cure we all hope and pray for
– Diana McGovern,
secretary, The Myelin Project

'Susie Cornell is a shining example of the belief
that the most important thing in combating any
handicap is to remain positive and fit'
– Anthea Turner,
GMTV, London

THE
COMPLETE
MS BODY
MANUAL

A handbook of effective treatment
for people with Multiple Sclerosis
and those who care for them

Susie Cornell
Founder of the MS Under Pressure Programme

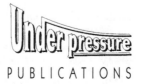

PUBLICATIONS

An UNDER PRESSURE PUBLICATION

© Susie Cornell 1996

First published in Great Britain in 1996 by
Under Pressure Publications
PO Box 1270
Chelmsford, CM2 6BQ, UK

Design and typesetting by Rainbow Greenheart
Illustrations by Nick Baxter
Cover by Wilf Preece
Printed and bound in Great Britain by
Fisher Print Services, Hailsham, East Sussex BN27 2BY, UK

British Library Cataloguing in Publication data available

ISBN 0 9527830 0 2

Contents

Acknowledgements

To the many people who have helped me in so many different ways I would like to say thank you. Thank you especially to the people who have believed and trusted in me, particularly all those who have come to me for help and guidance with MS and to the patients I have seen over the last five years who have willingly given their time to be a part of my MS therapy and research programme. I would not have been able to achieve anything without them and I hope they have benefited from the programme as much as I have benefited from helping them.

Thanks also to the Peto Institute in Hungary and the Foundation for Conductive Education in Birmingham, especially to Andrew Sutton who made it possible for me to attend the Institute in the first place and conductors Mel Brown and Aggi Mikula Toch who gave me the inspiration and determination to succeed; to Bryyon Lambert who shared his valuable insights into bio-engineering with me; to Dr Paul Sherwood who allowed me to study his unique approach to physical therapy; to the International Therapy Examinations Council (ITEC) for helping me to qualify as a professional therapist and tutor; to the MS campaigner Diana McGovern, secretary of the British Trust for the Myelin Project, who is always there when I need her; to John Simpkins of the MS Resource Centre, my local MS charity CHARMS and other MS organisations who have helped or supported me over the years; and to all the team at Under Pressure for their support and encouragement throughout.

For their help with this book thanks to Samantha Christie and Sue Lamming of Lamberts Healthcare (Nature's Best) for their invaluable nutritional input; to the health writer Richard Thomas for his priceless assistance in organising my material and showing me how to present it in a clear and readable way; to Nick Baxter for the illustrations, David Simpson for the design and production; and to Wilf Preece for the cover and photograph.

Thanks are also due to Anthea Turner for her constant support over many years; to my family and friends who have lived with my work and put up with me through the bad times as well as the good; to my nephew Ben, a sufferer from cerebral palsy, who was with me at the Peto Institute; and last, but by no means of course least, to my husband Ian for being there for me, supporting, cajoling, and encouraging so that I not only kept my eyes clearly on the vision but my feet firmly on the ground. I hope they all think it has been as worth while in the end as I do.

To Ian

Foreword

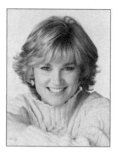

by Anthea Turner

Susie Cornell is a friend I have known for many years and who I admire greatly. Like many people, Susie discovered she had MS in the prime of her life with everything to live for and a lot of living still to do. That fighting spirit and zest never left her and in discovering ways to help her own condition, she set out to help others. This book is a result of that journey.

One of her main achievements is the unique and revolutionary health and fitness centre she has created in Essex with her husband Ian. Catering for all those many people who might otherwise be intimidated by the 'muscle-bound' environment usually found at such clubs, Under Pressure in Chelmsford is a model of friendliness and accessibility – where no one is put under any pressure if they don't want it!

Susie has not found a cure for MS – no one has – but she has discovered significant ways of improving the quality of life. She is a shining example of the belief that the most important thing in combating any handicap is to remain positive and fit.

After reading this book I hope you will be positive and fit too!

Anthea

GMTV London
June 1996

Preface

Dr Paul Sherwood *MB, BCh*

Best-selling author of *The Back and Beyond*, *The Heart Revolution* and *Asthma and Beyond*

I have been privileged to know Susie Cornell for several years now and have occasionally worked with her. She is an inspiration not only to all people with multiple sclerosis but also to doctors and other professional healthcarers she comes into contact with over the treatment of this distressing and disabling illness.

With so many intractable diseases like MS one finds views generally polarised between those who take the negative line – that the disease is incurable and sufferers cannot really be helped – and others with a more positive approach. This is the one which says that even though there may yet be no cure there is much that can be done to improve the quality of life of the people involved so let's do it.

The positive approach in MS is the one that says patients' quality of life can be greatly improved by helping them to cope better with the disease by understanding it, by using their bodies to the very best potential possible, by providing them with facilities that allow them to overcome many of their problems, and – from my own experience of treating people with MS – by giving them the physical therapy and exercises employed by Susie Cornell.

These exercises, developed by Susie very carefully and skilfully over many years of practical experience with her own disability and that of others, are not only of great value in helping people manage the effects of MS but also delay the progress of the disease and improve the patient's actual physical condition.

I cannot therefore recommend this book too highly to people with MS as well as to those involved in the care of people with MS, to relatives and friends of people who suffer and to the public at large – for all of whom it provides a wider and sympathetic understanding of where so much help in improving quality of life is possible but little is currently available.

Harley Street,
London, England.

Richard Thomas

Author of The Natural Way with MS

People, especially doctors, often ask me what qualifications non-doctors have for writing the sort of book Susie Cornell has here. By what right do 'amateurs' claim to offer the advice they do, say the 'professionals'? The hidden question, the one they really mean, of course, is what are non-doctors doing horning in on 'our' patch?

It is certainly true that Susie Cornell is not a doctor and has no formal medical qualifications. But the reply I give in specific examples such as this book is the reply Susie herself gives – and it is the best anyone can give in my opinion: she's been there, done it, and come through.

In other words, her qualifications are those of experience. She's not only lived with MS for more than 20 years but worked out exactly how to help herself in the most practical and positive way possible. Not many doctors can say that!

What is also important, though, is that Susie has not confined her discoveries to herself, as many might, but reached out to others to share her benefits with them – and give to them some of the positive spirit she radiates. For this she is only to be thanked and applauded as far as I'm concerned. Heaven knows the medical profession at large does little enough for people with MS.

That is why I am more than happy to support this book. It does not contain any mysterious secret or offer overnight 'miracle' cures from a cola bottle that build up hopes unrealistically one day only to see them dashed to the ground the next. It holds something much more precious for all those unfortunate enough to have MS: a wealth of sound, positive advice and information ladled out generously with that special seasoning that is Susie's uniquely optimistic style.

I know this is a book that will bring help and support to many and one of the most important ways it will do so is by lifting the spirits of all who read it with its message of hope. There are few more important things anyone in the field of healing can do – doctor or non-doctor. I wish Susie and all those with MS the best of luck in the world.

Shaftesbury,
Dorset, England.

An Introduction to the author

'The most infectious thing is a smile'

The saying above has been Susie's watchword for years now and nothing sums up her life and work better. A smile is a most infectious thing, indeed. Most people know it but few of them have had to overcome the problems Susie has and still believe in it. Smiling, though, is her trademark. No matter what life has thrown at her – and to date Susie's journey through life has been nothing if not difficult – she has always managed not only to keep smiling herself but to keep those around her smiling too.

I did not know Susie in her early years in Birmingham but those who did, her family most of all, tell me she was just the same then. Of course, she was not to know at that time that she would be struck down by MS by the time she was barely out of her teens but the remarkable thing about Susie is that even if she had known I doubt she would have been very different. Her positive attitude to life and her determination to succeed at all costs is an inspiration to all who know her. It is what attracted me to her in the first place and it is that same attitude that is now attracting those unfortunate enough, like her, to suffer from MS.

Who is this remarkable woman? Let me tell you just a little about her.

The early years

After grammar school, Susie's zest for life and her looks soon took her away from her first job as a secretary into fashion modelling. This was a career that demanded long hours and hard work as well as making punishing demands on the body from the constant dieting to retain that all-important figure. But at least there was the travelling and it was travel that took her next to Majorca.

A chance meeting with the American owner of the English-language commercial radio station in Palma led her to becoming a radio presenter and DJ. She took to her new career like a duck to water and her infectious personality on air soon earned her the nickname 'Birmingham Sue' from her many admiring listeners.

But that was only the start. As full of pioneering ideas as ever, she initiated one of the first phone-in request programmes on radio in Europe – and we are talking about the very early 1970s here – and was soon interviewing the long line of film stars and show business personalities that were then arriving in Majorca in large numbers. All that came to an abrupt end in 1974 when she was diagnosed as having MS. She was just 23.

Puzzling symptoms in her legs took her through a series of medical tests and, eventually, to the diagnosis of MS. To say she was shattered by the diagnosis is an understatement. Like many a person before her and since, she thought her world had come come to an end - and for a while indeed it did. But it is not in Susie's nature to admit defeat and once she had got over the intial shock she decided it was time to fight back.

The start of the search

Now started her long search to discover the hidden secrets of her debilitating illness so that she could start to do something about it. Her first disappointment was to discover that the medical profession, by and large, were of little help – except to offer advice on how to get hold of a wheelchair and incontinence pads! A doctor in Harley Street, Dr Douglas Latto, put Susie on a near-Vegan diet – something she had never dreamed of doing before – and, one by one, she tried all the known alternative therapies going, noting the benefits of each as she went.

When hyperbaric oxygen (HBO) became known as a possible treatment for MS, Susie was one of the first to become involved. She became a founding member of a local group raising money for an HBO chamber and trying the therapy enthusiastically herself. But, again, she found the benefits were short-lived.

By now her legs were badly affected so her search continued. Finally, in 1988, she became the first adult from Britain with MS to attend the now world-famous Peto Institute for Conductive Education in Budapest, Hungary. It was a turning point.

Susie spent two months in Budapest undergoing treatment and

digesting the unconventional philosophy behind the work of the Peto Institute.

According to the institute the body is there to be used and problems only start if it is not. So the staff at the institute – they call themselves 'conductors' – told Susie that in their opinion only 10 per cent of her legs problem was due to MS, the rest – 90 per cent – was from lack of use. They proceeded to put her through a strict programme of physical work (some of which experience she describes in this book) before acute homesickness brought her home.

Back in Britain again, Susie promptly put her new-found knowledge to good use. She started a series of exercise classes for people with MS at the local MS charity where she was involved and at a local hospital. Results were extraordinary, and as word spread demand for the exercises grew.

At about the same time she met an Australian 'bio-engineer' who introduced her to yet another new concept. This was the technique of using specialized weight resistance machinery.

The 'Under Pressure' clinic opens

The Hungarian Peto work combined with the Australian pressure technique was, needless to say, soon adapted to include exercises Susie had by now devised herself specifically for people with MS. The new combined programme was called 'MS Under Pressure' and it was at once introduced into the brand new health and therapy centre I had by now built close to Chelmsford canal specially for Susie called, naturally, 'Under Pressure'.

That was in 1993 and the work has raced ahead ever since.

Tireless and as full of ideas as ever, Susie has produced a video of her exercises so that anyone can benefit from her work no matter where in the world they live. She has trained in a range of natural therapies, including physical therapy, massage, sports injury therapy, aromatherapy, reflexology and nutrition and started her own school of natural therapies. And now there is this wonderful book!

Susie often said to me over the years how strange it was that whenever anyone bought a new car they got a manual with it to explain how it worked but that no manual ever came with an illness, and especially one such as MS. Well, now there is such a manual and this is it.

Typically, Susie has made sure it is one that explains to anyone any-where exactly what can be done to make sure that MS is not the feared and frightening disease that many people think it is. Also, that there is a very great deal indeed that can be done to alleviate many of its more unpleasant symptoms and side-effects.

I may say I am pleased to be a part of her work and, above all, to be her husband. It's hard work – but rewarding. And she still makes me smile!

Ian Cornell
Chelmsford, UK.

Introduction

Being diagnosed with MS changed my life forever. Suddenly the body I had taken for granted had broken down and I didn't know why.

I had total faith then in medical science and believed that it was only a matter of time before the experts would come up with a cure. But one day something happened that made me start to question those 'experts'.

It was late spring and I was watching my neighbour lovingly bend her faded daffodils over and tie them up with string. When I asked her why she was doing it she said that she had been told by experts that it would add goodness to the bulbs. I thought about this but could not see the logic of it at all. If nature had intended daffodils to be tied over in this way for their own good, I said to myself, surely nature would have given them string to do it with and arms to tie it up with as well!

Some years later experts announced that instead of tying daffodils they should be left, as I had in fact done to mine instinctively. Thus it was that I started to listen to and believe in my own intuition.

I began to read everything I could about MS and study as much as possible about the human body. I tried anything and everything that seemed as if it might help, from hyberbaric oxygen and special diets to homeopathy and exercises. All this experience led me to look 'holistically' at the treatment of MS. That is, to see MS not as a disease out there on its own, somehow independent of the person who has it, but as the symptom of a state of dis-ease within each individual in relation to the world as a whole.

The result is that I now see the human body as like a finely-tuned clock, each intricate working part in delicate balance with every other part so that it takes only the smallest movement or change or interference to upset the movement and slow the clock down or even stop it altogether. Seen another way I think we are like the earth we live on and on which we depend. The earth is 70 per cent water. So is the air that surrounds us – and so are we. Upset this crucial natural balance and a state of unbalance or 'dis-ease' results.

We usually get a manual when we buy a car – but not when we are born. The result is that I think most people go through their lives unconsciously looking for a manual that doesn't exist! Certainly I have spent half of my life trying to find a way of helping my body return to that state of balance (or 'homeostasis') that is health. This book, then, is the result of that search. This is my 'manual' for people with that state of dis–ease known as MS.

I hope that all those with MS reading this manual will be helped to discover for themselves ways of 'fine-tuning' this precious piece of machinery we call the human body so that they will be able, like me, to return to that all-important state of homeostasis and full health.

Susie Cornell
Chelmsford, UK
June 1996

Special note for those in wheelchairs

Although many of the physical exercises in this book appear not to be suitable for people in wheelchairs, in fact, with assistance, all are suitable for anyone with MS, whether or not they are wheelchair-bound.

1 So you think you've got...

ms

You think you've got multiple sclerosis (MS) because your vision is a bit blurred or you have some tingling in your hands or feet and you've read somewhere that those are symptoms of MS.

It's true, those are symptoms of MS – but having them does not mean you have MS. There are a whole range of conditions that can produce all those symptoms and more, and all of which are treatable. In fact the probability is that you are much more likely to have something else entirely such an acute case of stress, tense neck muscles or a trapped nerve.

I have seen many, many people in my more than 20 years of having MS myself and dealing with people who have MS and I can tell you that a significant proportion of those who come to me thinking they might have MS don't have it at all. Their symptoms are the result of something else that can be treated and overcome very easily and effectively.

Lynn is just one example, although a particularly dramatic one. A fit and active 58-year-old still heavily involved in helping to run a family business, she came to me one sunny summer's day in 1994 in a totally distraught state. She had pains in her head, blurred vision and tingling in her left arm. Her specialist had just told her she had MS.

The first thing she did was burst into tears in front of me. Her daughter, who had brought her, told me privately her mother was so desperate she was concerned for her safety and sanity.

I spoke to Lynn quietly for a while and asked her a lot of questions. From what she was telling me I soon began to doubt that she had MS. With all the experience I have had in dealing with people with MS the right bells just weren't ringing for me and I was not fully convinced.

For one thing I knew it is unusual for anyone to contract MS at her age. The next thing I did was to feel around the back of her neck, especially what are known as the upper trapezius muscles supporting the neck. I was surprised to find how restricted her neck movement was. Something told me that here might be the real cause of her problem.

Sure enough, after only a couple of treatments at my centre in Chelmsford, just outside London, her symptoms all improved dramatically. The tingling in her arm went, her vision improved and so did the pains in her head.

Two treatments later she went to see a new specialist, another neurologist. Immediately after seeing him she rang me in a state of near ecstasy: the neurologist had told her she didn't have MS after all!

By one of life's extraordinary coincidences I ran into Lynn two years later in the middle of a busy London store. She saw me first and I remember hearing this voice calling out my name across a sea of heads. I looked around and there was Lynn rushing towards me, arms out and a huge smile on her face, ready to give me a big hug. When we disentangled she told me she had never had a chance to thank me properly for giving her back her life, as she put it.

Other examples are only a little less dramatic and illustrate my belief that many people who think they have MS may not at all. For example Connie, a 61-year-old grandmother and the wife of a retired local company secretary, came to see me after six years of suffering from what she had been told by her doctors was MS.

Her symptoms were pains in her legs and eyesight so bad she had been officially registered blind. Moorfields Hospital in London, one of the world's top eye hospitals, had told her there was nothing more they could do for her. She must face a life with severely limited vision, able to see only the blurred shapes of people and objects, they told her.

Connie described it to me as like trying to see through a dirty window with a big smudge in the middle!

We began working on her neck, the muscles of her back and manipulating her spine. After a few months of us doing this twice a week Connie began to notice a very definite improvement in her eyesight. The first thing she realized was that she could read all the car number plates in the park outside the centre. Then she found she could see the time on the clock in the exercise area.

Today she regards her eyesight as 'at least 25 per cent improved on what it was.' Not bad for someone top eye specialists had said nothing could be done! (Her story is told in more detail in chapter 3.)

Although it has not been established beyond doubt I think it may still turn out that Connie's problem is not MS at all. I think the problem with her eyes is more the result of fibrositis in her neck and her leg pains are the result of a virtual lifetime of digestive disorders and a 'weak bladder'. This was almost confirmed for me later, shortly before this book went to press, when Connie had to get urgent medical attention for a blocked bowel.

Another case is Barbara, a 34-year-old hairdresser. As well as blurred and double vision with pain behind her eyes, she was in so much agony each time she bent over she could no longer carry on working. Pins and needles and numbness in her working hand were further problems.

She had been diagnosed with MS in 1992, five years after her first symptoms and two years before coming to see me. Just two treatment sessions on her neck – each session an intensive half hour – were enough to give her what she described to me at the time as 'immediate relief.' All the pains in her head went – and so far have never come back.

This was with a woman who had been told by doctors she had major damage to her brain stem and, again, there was nothing they could do to improve the pains. The pains, they said, would probably never be any better.

Barbara is now back at work as a hairdresser and has no further problems – though she still comes in every three or four weeks for therapy to her neck (which I'll write more about a little later).

All these women thought they had MS – and so, it must be said, did their doctors. But what I think is far more likely is that their symptoms were the result of some basic, and probably long-standing, neck problem.

Stiffness and congestion in the neck area is just one of the simple problems that can cause symptoms similar to MS and can be just as easily put right with massage and manipulation. Another is faulty eating habits and a poor diet.

For example, many of the symptoms of MS, I am convinced after years of research and experience, relate to a lack of the right balance of nutrients in your body – that is, to a deficiency of vitamins, minerals and amino acids.

A lack of manganese in the diet of children, for instance, can commonly cause growing pains. That's what happened to me. From the age of about eight to the age of 10 I suffered considerable growing pains – so much so I would wake up in the night crying with the agony of it and my mother would sit up massaging my legs for me to get me to go back to sleep.

Because the doctor said it was due to lack of exercise my mother took me to dancing lessons. But in fact I now know the pains were all due to a simple manganese deficiency.

The same deficiency in an adult can cause insomnia, restlessness, aches and pains in the back and joints, lack of energy, lack of sex drive, dizziness, muscle twitches, muscles spasms, balance problems and pains in the knees.

Chemical pollution is yet another suspect in the mystery of MS. Ben, a West Country sheep farmer in his mid 40s, came to see me in 1994 after being officially diagnosed with MS in 1991, two years into suffering constant numbness in his fingertips.

The diagnosis was made by a neurologist, a nerve specialist, following a scan by a Magnetic Resonance Imager (MRI), the latest technology for diagnosing MS. On the basis of the scan the neurologist said he felt Ben 'almost certainly had MS' in spite of the fact that he noted that Ben also had some curvature of his lower spine and disc protrusions in his neck.

By the time I saw him, Ben had blurred vision in both eyes, numbness in both hands and an 'inconsistent' bladder – but he still said his biggest problem was his back. A further complication was that for years he had been working with sheep-dip, a liquid for 'de-lousing' sheep. Sheep-dip contains *organophosphates*, poisonous chemicals now known to cause serious damage to the nerves in humans and sometimes leading to death.

Ben's symptoms are very similar to those experienced by other farmers known to be affected by organophosates but, surprisingly, Ben told me his specialist had made no mention of the fact that he is far more likely to be suffering from pesticide poisoning from the sheep-dip than MS.

It is still unclear whether Ben actually has MS, even though that is what he and his doctors now think. Even more surprising to me, though, is the way his spinal problems have apparently been dismissed. I think it is far more likely that Ben's symptoms are more to do with pesticide poisoning and spinal problems than MS and that he does not have MS at all. Time will tell.

What these stories show is not only just how difficult and uncertain diagnosis is with MS but also how powerful a factor the mind is in the treatment of disease. The mind is a very potent trigger of so many things and its part in MS – especially the part played by stress and mental and emotional traumas of all sorts – is, I believe, beyond doubt.

Other causes of MS – or rather the symptoms given the name MS – are, in my experience, physical injuries (such as whiplash), viral infections and persistent throat infections. All the people mentioned so far have suffered from at least one or more of these problems before they were diagnosed with MS.

I'll tell you more about these findings later, but what they have done is to lead me to question much of what doctors know and say about MS – and I include the very name 'MS' in this.

■ The 'MS' label

The very first thing I often say to anyone who thinks they might have MS is to forget the name. Just being told 'Oh, you have MS' can seem almost like a death sentence to some people. They latch onto the name and their world falls apart!

I know how such people feel because I felt exactly the same way – and for a long time my world did fall apart.

For years I suffered in isolation as the doctors all told me they could do nothing. My whole life was wrapped up in MS. I couldn't do anything because I had MS. I was a prisoner to MS. I felt every cough and every cold, every ache and every pain was MS. The doctors told me it was MS and naturally I believed them. I believed everything they told me in those days.

But my objection to the MS label is not just down to the mental and emotional damage it can cause. I actually think MS is an inappropriate name to give the condition.

'Multiple sclerosis' sounds so medical, so definite, doesn't it? But it means nothing much at all really. 'Multiple' means 'a lot' and 'sclerosis' is from an ancient Greek word meaning 'hard'. So 'multiple sclerosis' is simply a fancy name for 'a great deal of hardened or scarred tissue'. Not very specific when you get down to it, is it?

So what is 'MS' deep down? Well, officially of course it is damage to the myelin sheath, the fatty tissue surrounding nerve fibres. This then affects the central nervous system because the signals that run through the nerve fibres get distorted or interrupted so the brain doesn't get the right message.

But this doesn't really tell us anything about what is behind MS. What causes it in the first place, for example?

I believe the answer lies in a breakdown of the immune system caused by malabsorption and maldigestion *(See Appendix B, 'The leaky gut' connection)*. Clearly there does seem to be something with the genetic makeup of some people that makes them more prone to getting MS than others but even so my feeling is that it still needs something extra to push those people 'over the brink', as it were.

This something extra could be, as I've already said, many things – wrong diet, nutritional and digestive enzyme deficiency, throat infections, physical injury, emotional trauma and stress, environmental pollution – and it can lead just as easily to a whole range of illnesses and problems, some serious, others very minor. MS is just one of them.

So the first thing I'd say to anyone who thinks they may have MS is to forget the label. Throw it out of the window. MS can only be properly diagnosed after extensive medical tests and even then, as most doctors will admit, diagnosis is uncertain. So always think the best first. Consider that you probably don't have MS. Like a lot of people, you have a body that is out–of–balance. That's all.

Yes, I agree the symptoms are sometimes pretty awful but it isn't the end of the world. Look for other causes first. As I've proved, plenty of things can be done about it. It's what a lot of this book is about. For example, the immune system – in anyone – can be strengthened and boosted. An immune system imbalance can often be corrected and put right as a result.

That means symptoms resulting from such an imbalance can be considerably helped and allieviated. That applies as much to MS as to colds and 'flu, probably the commonest 'disorders' of the immune system.

What is the immune system?

The immune system is the special mechanism the body has for fighting threats to your health. If the nervous system is the body's 'telecommunications system', relaying messages to and fro between the brain and the muscles via the spinal cord, the immune system can be seen as part of the 'maintenance department', keeping the equipment in good repair.

In a normally healthy person the immune system is at work the whole time like an army of soldiers on constant watch, defending you against anything that might hurt or harm you, whether it is a virus, bacteria or some other 'invader'.

For something so important your body's immune system is really very simple. It consists basically of your blood supply and small sets of organs such as the thymus gland, lymph nodes and the spleen. The diagram on page 9 shows the whole system clearer.

Defense against disease is essentially a function of the white cells in blood and it is one of the jobs of this group of organs to produce these white cells, known as *leukocytes.*

White blood cells produce substances that defend the body against attack from anything harmful such as a virus. These defending substances are known as *antibodies* (attacking substances are known as *antigens*).

Looked at as a whole blood in our body is made up of roughly
- 40% red cells (known as *erythrocytes*) and

■   60% plasma, a semi-clear mixture of proteins (including vitamins) and mineral salts. A very small amount is made up of the white cells (leukocytes) that I've already mentioned, and special clotting agents called *platelets*. Other ingredients include the hormones that are the body's vital 'chemical controllers', controlling your essential activities.

Blood is made mainly in bone marrow (especially the long bones of the ribs, backbone, breastbone, thighbones and skull) but also in the lymph nodes and spleen. All red blood cells and some white cells come from bone marrow but white cells are also produced by the lymph nodes and the spleen.

White cells are the really important cells in fighting disease and they come in three main types:

■   macrophages
■   bone-marrow cells (known as B cells)
■   thymus cells (T cells).

Macrophages are large cells – seen through a miscroscope they are a mixture of round and elongated shapes – and are the major fighting cells. They are the 'cleaners-up'. They surround and 'hoover up' any harmful substance such as a virus (as well as the defending antibodies) before disposing of everything through the lymphatic system.

B-cells make the substance that destroys an attacking substance. They also have a memory that can recognise and attack past attacking substances.

T-cells are split into 'T helpers' and 'T suppressors' and both are needed to keep the immune system balanced. T-cells contain chemicals called *cytotoxins* that kill infected cells and make a virus-blocking protein called *interferon* (the new MS drugs such as Beta-interferon are a synthetic version of it).

Though the immune system is cleverly programmed to be able to tell what is good and what bad for the body – so it will reject only the bad things – sometimes this programming goes wrong. Normally the immune system only fails when it is so overloaded with the strength of an attack, such as a particularly strong virus,

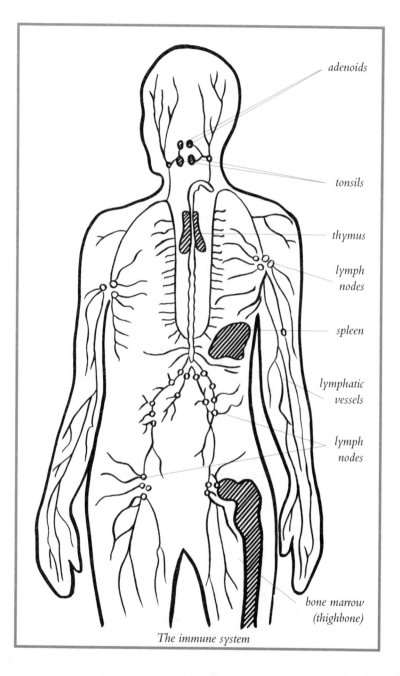

adenoids

tonsils

thymus

lymph nodes

spleen

lymphatic vessels

lymph nodes

bone marrow (thighbone)

The immune system

the attacking agents win – at least until the immune system has had time to muster its defenders and mount a successful counter-attack. This is what happens in 'flu, for example.

But there are times when the system breaks down and for various reasons the defenders turn against the body instead of defending it. Illnesses resulting when this happens are called 'auto-immune diseases'. Examples include allergies (where the immune system overreacts to normally harmless substances such as animal hair or pollen) and Aids. Many doctors these days think MS may be another.

For me, it is very important to consider what else may be causing the symptoms complained of before accepting the MS diagnosis – even those who have been officially diagnosed.

If it's a surprise that I'm questioning the official diagnosis of MS by a trained and qualified medical practitioner it really shouldn't be. Doctors are the first to know they are not infallible and the truth is that MS is very hard to diagnose accurately, even with quite sophisticated equipment. Even Magnetic Resonance Image (MRI) scanning, considered the latest and best diagnostic tool for MS, is now known to be not as accurate in detecting damage to myelin sheath as it was once thought to be.

However at the end of the day it is possible that you do, in fact, like me, have myelin sheath damage and what is called 'MS'. If that applies to you it's time to start working on the many things you can do to alleviate the symptoms to their maximum. In the rest of this book I'll tell you more about MS and exactly how to go about managing it.

2 You've been diagnosed with...

ms

If you are one of those who has undergone tests for MS and been told by doctors you definitely have MS don't despair. Still look for more obvious reasons for the symptoms.

As I've already said in the previous chapter, even if someone has been to their doctor and been officially diagnosed as 'having MS' they should still look to other explanations first. The diagnosis may still be open to debate. I've seen any number of people who have been told they had MS that I have then discovered didn't have MS at all. That's why the first thing I do whenever anyone comes to me saying they have MS is check their diagnosis and symptoms. Of course examples of this are uncommon but they are by no means rare I can assure you!

But even if you are in that category of people who probably do have MS – that is, their symptoms are the result of damage to the myelin sheath around their main nerve fibres – you can be helped far more than you realise.

Take the example of Anne. Anne came to me at 49 in 1993 after having been officially diagnosed with MS the year before. Her symptoms were a pain in her left eye which she described as 'like a knife being twisted'. She had had this 'unbearable' pain consistently for ten years – but had only been diagnosed after she'd been to see her doctor with tingling in her hands and legs and some numbness in her face.

In Anne's case I felt, after talking to her, she had been correctly diagnosed – but over a period of time of receiving my treatment, which included work on her spine and especially neck as well as advice on diet and lifestyle, all her symptoms subsided to the point that I feel her condition has now been stabilised.

Put another way, she now only comes to see me every three months instead of every week!

Causes of MS

I'd like to say a word or two at this point about the causes of MS. Basically the official line is that no one knows what causes MS – which is why there are almost as many theories as there are people with MS! I have done some research on this and the way I believe MS develops is that a combination of factors all have to come together in a certain way over a set period of time.

In sequence it looks something like this:

- A genetic weakness (or 'predisposition' as the doctors call it)
- A long-term nutritional deficiency or imbalance (possibly due to malabsorption)
- A long-term situation of emotional stress or strain (possibly coupled with a very specific emotional trauma)
- A severe infection, particularly of the throat (such as tonsillitis or glandular fever)
- A physical trauma or injury (this could be something dramatic such as whiplash but it could just as easily be something as simple and non-specific as falling off a chair: these sort of minor injuries often go undiagnosed and untreated because there is little or no pain and so the person injured this way doesn't think of it as an injury).

Often it is the emotional and physical trauma together that is the straw that almost literally breaks the person's back and brings on the first symptoms of MS. In my own case I remember when I was 17 I was out riding one day when I suddenly felt my spine 'give way'. It arched involuntarily in a way I couldn't control. At the time I was just getting over a very severe emotional trauma, the breakup of a relationship, and was also dieting very severely because of my modelling career. Two years later I had my first symptoms of MS.

The pattern I see in my own case I have now noticed in many others. With Anne, for example, I am sure that one of the most important triggers of her symptoms was a very severe whiplash injury she got in a car crash when she was 25. She also told me that in her late thirties she had suffered severe emotional stress followed by glandular fever and shingles.

Other examples are just as typical. Take the following three male patients of mine:

■ Derek, a 42-year-old former business manager for a large distribution company, had experienced both growing pains and severe throat infections and sinusitis consistently throughout his childhood. His business career put him under constant mental and emotional strain and in 1974, the year his first symptoms appeared, he suffered two serious footballing injuries. In 1984, two years before his official diagnosis, he had a severe bout of salmonella poisoning.

■ Former Royal Marine Tim was officially diagnosed in 1993 at 27, six years after he experienced his first symptoms. He had had a severe bout of tonsillitis at the age of 12, followed three years later by the deaths of his mother, uncle and grandfather – all within a few months of each other. A few years later, during his time as a marine, he had suffered damage to his spine during a practice parachute jump.

■ Nigel, a former senior officer in the Metropolitan Police in London, was not diagnosed until 1992 when he was 43, though his first symptoms appeared in 1975. As a young child he had had three bouts of very severe tonsillitis and very bad catarrh throughout his teens. Always athletic, involved in a number of sports, he had suffered a serious back and shoulder injury in 1965 doing judo. In 1974, the year before the appearance of his first symptoms, he underwent a highly stressful period at work resulting in him neglecting his eating so much that he admits his diet was completely inadequate.

My case file is full of similar examples – though, strangely, doctors I've told about my results don't seem very interested. The result was that in 1994 I decided to put my idea to the test. I carried out a very thorough survey of 40 people with MS and compared them with another 40 who didn't. What I found was very interesting indeed.

These are the results, published in 1996 in the *International Journal of Alternative & Complementary Medicine*:

	Group with MS	Group without MS
Incidence of throat infections	75%	25%
Physical injury	75%	25%
Viral infection	70%	30%
Emotional trauma	60%	40%
Poor diet and lifestyle	60%	40%

Following on from this I now believe that the following five key factors (apart, that is, from genetic predisposition or having 'MS genes') are common to everyone who has MS:

- persistent throat infections that start in early childhood
- some sort of back injury – such as a car accident, sports injury or major fall – at some stage in life
- a serious viral infection having happened at some point, such as penumonia, glandular fever or hepatitis
- some serious emotional trauma having happened at some stage also – for example, a divorce, bereavement or redundancy
- having a poor diet and leading an unhealthy lifestyle over a long period.

Taking a case history

Now, as a result of these conclusions, when anyone comes to see me I sit them down and go through a detailed questionnaire that tells me several vital things I need to know about their past and medical history. For example, as well as their age, date of birth, date of first symptoms and diagnosis, I ask them:

- if they had any traumas or difficulties when they were born
- if they had throat infections at any stage
- if they have ever had tonsillitis and whether or not they still have their tonsils
- if they had any growing pains as a child

- if they have ever had problems with their sinuses
- if they have ever had asthma or any other chest problems or infections
- if they have ever had any serious illness or illnesses, and if so what and when
- if they have ever had any emotional trauma or upset in their lives and when
- if they have ever had any accidents, injuries or falls and when
- if they have ever had any unexplained sensations in their back or spine at any time
- if they have ever suffered from dietary deficiency at any stage in their lives and when
- if there is any history of genetic weakness of any sort in their family
- if there is any history of MS in their family at all
- if their parents are still living.

The answers to these questions alone give me a pretty good idea of who can be helped and to what degree. Some questions, such as the ones on diet and nutrition for example, are quite complex and take some time to go into, but thanks to the latest testing procedures I use I can find out a lot about someone's nutritional status without the need for lengthy questioning via hair mineral analysis, a special way of testing by analysing a sample of hair chemically .

This first questionnaire is followed by another in which I ask patients to tell me of any medical conditions they may have or be aware of that could affect their treatment such as migraine, epilepsy, high blood pressure or diabetes.

Following the questionnaires and nutritional status test, each patient has a full physical assessment that measures their muscular strength, dexterity and coordination. This assessment is something I have developed over some years and is unlike any tests done anywhere else.

It is followed by a physical check of the person's spinal column and the muscles surrounding it to discover any other possible problems that might lie behind the symptoms experienced.

What is MS?

For those not entirely sure of exactly what, medically speaking, MS is let me tell you. MS is the breakdown of myelin, a sort of fatty tissue, that surrounds nerve fibres in the body like insulation around electrical wiring. This 'insulating' tissue is called 'myelin sheath'. (Myelin sheath also makes the initials MS so hence another, unofficial, way of describing MS as 'myelin sheath disease'.)

What happens in MS is that some fault in the way the body works causes this fatty tissue to become randomly inflamed and this in turn causes the covering to become pitted and scarred where the inflammation has taken place. This hardened scarring interferes with the way that the signals that pass along the nerve fibres send messages to the brain. The result is that the right messages don't reach the brain and so the brain can't send the correct messages to the parts of the body controlled by certain nerves *(see diagram opposite)*.

Note: Though many people think MS is a disease of the muscles it is not. There is nothing at all wrong with the muscles of people with MS, they are perfectly healthy. They don't work properly because they aren't getting the right messages, that's all. This information is very important in the treatment of MS, as we'll see.

Treating MS

Most of this book is taken up with explaining the treatment of MS by the parts of the body most affected. There are two reasons for this. The first is to make it simple for people with problems with their eyes or legs or wherever to find what can help them quickly and easily on the basis of their most obvious symptoms. But the other reason is because the nervous system and various parts of the body as well as important organs within the body are all intimately linked in very particular ways.

The two major diagrams on pages 18 and 19 – which are more detailed versions of the simplified illustration of the nervous system opposite – hopefully explain it better than any words of mine. The

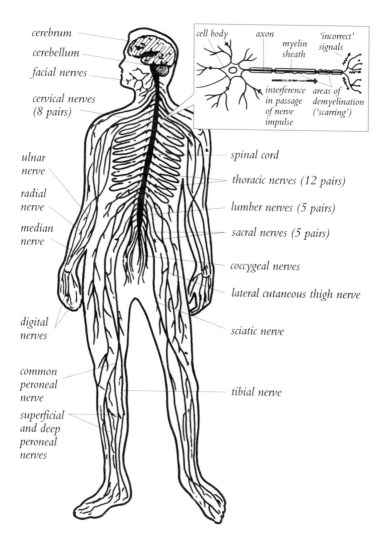

*The central nervous system and
(inset) an individual nerve fibre affected by MS*

first diagram shows how all the vital organs of the body are connected by the nerves to the spinal cord, the main 'power cable' that runs directly from the brain down through the centre of the backbone (or spine), and the second how nerves run from the spine to the various extremities of the body.

The really important part of both diagrams is seeing which areas of the spinal cord and the spine connect to which organ and part of the body. So, for example, in the first diagram (below) different parts of the spinal cord deal with two different, though complementary, parts

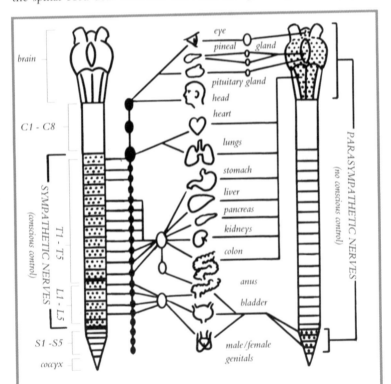

Schematic diagram of the autonomic nervous system.

The sympathetic nerves (left) connect to the body organs via the vertebral ganglion, while the parasympathetic nerves (right) connect to the organs from the opposite ends of the spinal chord.

of the *autonomic nervous system* (autonomic means it controls automatic functions like breathing, digesting, seeing and so on).

The 'sympathetic' nervous system, which covers the organs that control most of the basic essential functions of life such as our heart, lungs, digestive system, bladder, bowels and so on, is situated in the middle part of the spinal cord. The 'parasympathetic' nervous system, which is concerned mainly with the functions of the brain and genitals, is split on the other hand between the top and bottom ends of the spinal cord. Note that the top end of the spinal cord is in the brain itself.

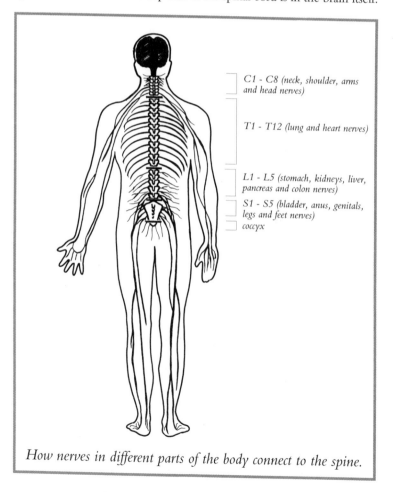

C1 - C8 *(neck, shoulder, arms and head nerves)*

T1 - T12 *(lung and heart nerves)*

L1 - L5 *(stomach, kidneys, liver, pancreas and colon nerves)*

S1 - S5 *(bladder, anus, genitals, legs and feet nerves)*

coccyx

How nerves in different parts of the body connect to the spine.

The schematic diagram on page 18 can be usefully related to the illustration on the previous page showing how the the nerves connect to the spine. Note how the nerves radiate out from four distinct part of the spine to cover four distinct parts of the body:

■ The top eight spinal bones *(vertebrae)* (C1–C8) deal with the neck, shoulders, arms and hands.

■ The next twelve bones (T1–T12) cover the heart and lungs

■ The third set (L1–L5) connect to the stomach, kidneys, liver, pancreas and colon

■ The bottom set (S1–S5, excluding the 'tail bone' or coccyx) are responsible for the bladder, genitals and anus as well as legs and feet.

It is easy to see from these diagrams why neck and lower back problems feature so heavily in so many of today's illnesses and also how they relate to many of the symptoms of MS. I'll go into these in more detail in later chapters but let me explain a bit more at this point about what I do when someone comes to me who I think probably does have a problem of demyelination (and therefore 'classic' MS).

What happens next ?

I always treat people individually according to their symptoms. So the next step, after the tests, is to look particularly at how well each person's immune system is working. I also look at their diet and lifestyle, their exercise routine and breathing habits.

Checking the immune system

Checking the immune system is the first and most important thing for anyone with MS. Anyone can check on the health of their immune system by doing a few simple tests such as the ones suggested by Jennifer Meek in her excellent book *Immune Power* (Optima, UK, 1990).

For example, do you notice any of the following:

■ Hair

Does your hair fall out? Is it greasy or dry? Do you suffer from dandruff?

■ Head

Do you suffer from dull aches in your head, or foggy, floaty, dizzy feelings? Do you feel sharp pains in your head, or pains on moving or behind the eyes? Do you suffer from flushing or burning sensations in your face?

■ Eyes

Are the whites of your eyes yellowed or blood-shot? Do your eyes suffer from twitching, or feel itchy, scratchy or watery? Do you get a dull pain in your eyes when you move them from side to side? Do you get blurred or impaired vision? Do your eyes feel tired?

■ Ears

Do you get noises inside your ears? Do they feel 'bubbly' inside? Do they itch, is the skin flakey and do they hurt?

■ Nose

Do you suffer from loss of smell, difficulty breathing, mucus, a running nose, itching nose, sneezing, a sore nose?

■ Mouth

Do you suffer from mouth ulcers, bad breath, bleeding gums, loss of taste, a coated tongue, difficulty in chewing, lack of saliva?

■ Neck

Do you suffer from a stiff neck or pain on moving your neck?

■ Throat

Do you suffer from swollen or painful glands, an itching or sore throat, or do you have difficulty swallowing?

■ Digestive system

Do you suffer from indigestion, wind, a feeling of burning, being bloated or pain in the intestines, constipation or diarrhoea?

■ Muscles

Do you suffer from weak, painful, numb, tingling, flabby, tense, easily injured, jumping or twitching muscles?

■ Joints

Do you suffer from stiff, weak, swollen or painful joints?

■ Nails

Are your nails ridged, brittle, show white spots on them, split easily, have a blue tinge to them?

■ Energy levels

Are your energy levels high, low, erratic, or are you hyperactive?

■ Physical symptoms

Is your physical energy high, low, short-lived, dependent on taking food, drink or stimulants of various kinds?

■ Mental symptoms

Do you suffer from poor concentration, memory problems/ forgetfulness, and a general lack of interest in the world?

■ Mood changes

Do you feel constantly depressed, elated, sad, happy, irritable, frustrated, unstable? Do you have cravings for certain foods and/or drinks or feel hooked on them?

According to Jennifer Meek, positive answers to any of these questions mean you have an immune system that is under threat and needs active help and support to prevent it going over the edge.

Though this help and support varies, depending on which part of the body is affected, many of the methods I recommend – such as eating and breathing properly and the exercises summarised in Appendix A – are good for the immune system as a whole. In the following chapters, however, I'll describe them grouped under the symptoms they are usually most useful for based on my own experience in treating people with MS over the last ten years.

You'll find not only special exercises for people with MS you've probably never been told about before but advice on diet (or food) supplements that you'll probably never have heard of before either.

eyes

Believe it or not, a problem with your eyes may actually not be your eyes at all but your neck and shoulders. The sort of eye symptoms associated with MS – blurred or double vision, pain in the eyes or just a plain ache – are not only the result of the process of demyelination that technically leads to the condition known as MS. They are more often the result simply of stress and consequent tension in the neck muscles. So the first thing to do if you have a problem with your eyes is to check for non-MS causes such as 'stiff' neck.

■ Checking for non-MS causes of eye problems

I've found over the years that restricted neck movement is a classic feature of many of those with vision problems. So feeling and massaging someone's neck and shoulder muscles is often one of the first things I do when someone comes to see me. I've found that I can usually get a very good idea of someone's tension levels just by touching their neck in this way.

What has happened is that tension over the years has 'locked' their muscles into a

Treating eye problems
My treatments for eye problems consist of the following three approaches:
• Physical therapy
• Dietary and nutritional support
• Reflexology

hard inflexible mass and this has had a knock-on effect on other parts of the body, including affecting their vision. Double-vision and blurred vision are, of course, symptoms of MS – but they can also be caused by factors, such as 'solid neck' that have nothing to do with MS.

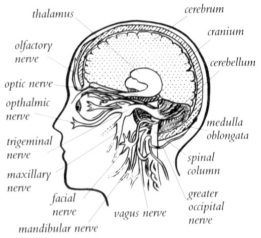

Nerves of the head and eyes

Even in cases of genuine MS, I have found that regular massage and manipulation of the neck and shoulders can produce quite astonishing benefits. In fact eye problems can be helped by the same sort of treatments whatever the cause.

Physical therapy

Manipulating or massaging what physical therapists call the 'soft tissue' – the muscles and sinews – of the neck and shoulders is an easy and, in my experience, highly effective way of helping with problems of vision and the head, such migraine and headaches, and not just those caused by MS.

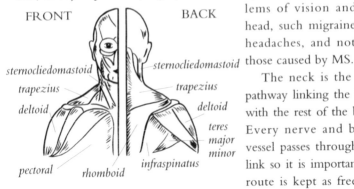

The neck muscles

The neck is the only pathway linking the brain with the rest of the body. Every nerve and blood vessel passes through this link so it is important the route is kept as free and uncongested as possible.

Congestion of any sort can quickly cause the sort of chaos you get on any main highway in the rush-hour!

Causes of congestion are both physical and psychological. Carrying heavy loads or an accident such as whiplash can give the neck a 'traffic jam' but so also can tension.

Tension is one of life's most underrated and insidious problems. It can be both the cause and effect of illness. In chronic form it can creep up on us unrecognized over months or even years and we finally only notice it when it starts giving us pain.

Coping with someone at work or at home we think is 'a pain in the neck' or holding back tears and fears can cause contractions of the muscles and changes in our pattern of breathing. Tense and stressful situations make our heart rate go up and our breathing become faster or they make us hold our breath and we 'freeze'. All this adds to the stress.

Driving is a classic cause of tension leading to neck strain. Have you ever noticed how sometimes when you drive you find yourself gripping the steering wheel tightly and clenching your teeth for no apparent reason? It is not until you've sat back in your seat and consciously relaxed that you realize how tense you were!

Tension interferes with the circulation of blood and lymph – both essential parts of our body's fighting mechanism against disease – and can restrict joint mobility. Restricted mobility can pull the body out of alignment, thus causing further and perhaps more serious mobility problems.

It is important when dealing with neck problems, particularly those caused by tension, to know that the muscles that attach the head to the upper body pass through the neck and then fan out into the back of the shoulders. So treating the neck shouldn't be done without 'warming up' the upper back and shoulders as well.

How is this done? Quite simply by massaging your neck and shoulder muscles yourself – or preferably getting someone else to massage you – and by practising neck muscle-stretching exercises.

Self massage

Begin by gently stroking down the side of your neck and across the shoulder. Keep the shoulders, hands and fingers relaxed and the palms moulded to the contours of the body.

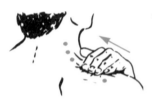

Self-help neck massage

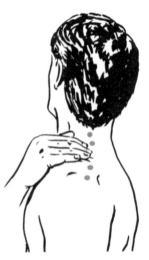

Then knead the shoulders by squeezing the muscle at the top of each shoulder between palm and fingers. This may feel quite tender, especially if there is tension in the shoulders, so go gently at first but continue kneading, looking particularly for areas or 'knots' of tautness, and the tenderness will pass.

If you find an area that is tender, hold it firmly and circle your shoulders first backwards and then forwards allowing the movement of the shoulder to do its own massage. You will feel the muscle stretching and relaxing.

Getting a friend to help

Start in a sitting position, not lying down. Get the friend to stand behind you and place their hands gently on both shoulders, a hand on either side. Begin with what is called effleurage. This is a light stroking movement that should start at the top of the neck and run slowly down the neck and out across the shoulders, hands relaxed and flat on the skin.

Without taking the hands off return the hands to the base of the neck with the fingers pointing towards the skull, making the whole exercise a circular movement. Repeat the move-

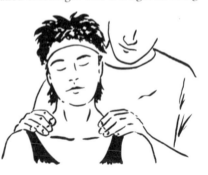

Neck massage from a friend

ment four or five times to relax the shoulders. Squeeze the top of the shoulders gently between palms and fingers and then finish with more gentle effleurage (stroking) movements.

Muscle-stretching exercises for the neck and shoulders

The results achieved by the manipulation above can be greatly enhanced and reinforced by special muscle-stretching exercises taught to all physical therapists (who call them 'soft tissue release exercises'). They, too, are relatively simple and once learnt from an experienced practitioner can be easily and effectively done at home. I have started many people off this way myself – and many of them have told me it's the first time they've had their necks touched, let alone stretched!

I have found a combination of the following exercises, done in sequence, are most effective. Altogether they shouldn't take more than about ten minutes and can be done at any time and anywhere.

■ Exercise 1

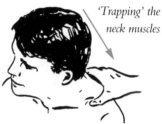
'Trapping' the neck muscles

Move your head over towards one shoulder and press down firmly on that shoulder with your fingers, so 'trapping' the large trapezius muscle in place at its furthest point from the neck (see right). Now slowly move your head over towards the other shoulder as far as it will go, keeping the muscle under pressure the whole time. You will feel it gently stretch as you move your head over. Repeat the procedure several times moving your fingers a little nearer the neck in small steps each time. You will find it

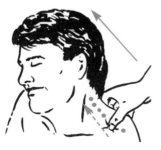

gets harder and harder to move your head right over to the opposite side the nearer the pressure on the trapezius muscle gets to your neck. This is normal but persevere with the stretch anyway. Repeat the procedure in a fan-like pattern across the back as far as the backbone. Now repeat the whole exercise on the opposite shoulder.

■ Exercise 2

Sit in an upright chair with your feet flat on the floor and your knees in line with your hips. Take a few deep breaths and shrug your shoulders a few times to relax. Turn your head slowly to the left as if looking over your left shoulder. Do the same to the right. Take your time, it is important not to strain.

■ Exercise 3

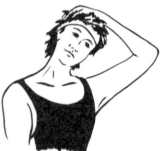

Now tuck your chin in and lower your ear towards your left shoulder. Hold this position. To increase the stretch bring your left hand to rest on the top of your head, fingertips towards your right ear (see diagram right). Relax and hold the position, allowing the weight of your hand and arm to increase the stretch. gradually. Repeat the exercise on the right side (right ear to right shoulder and so on).

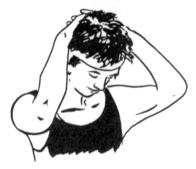

■ Exercise 4

Tuck your chin in and hold it there for a few seconds, feeling the stretch between your shoulder blades. Return your head to its normal position. Do it again but this time clasp your hands together behind your head and place them on the back of your head. Without pulling on your head, bring your elbows together towards your face, arms relaxed.

■ Exercise 5

Sitting in an upright position, breathe out and at the same time tilt your pelvis forward. Your back should now be rounded and your stomach muscles pulled in. Breathe in and return to a normal upright sitting position. To stretch further, tilt your pelvis forward

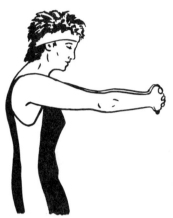

as before but this time with your arms out straight in front of you. Clasp your hands together and you should feel a stretch between your shoulder blades. Hold this for a few seconds and return to the upright position.

■ Exercise 6

Sitting in an upright position, place your hands behind you and hold the back of the chair. Now stretch your back by lifting your chest upwards towards the ceiling, neck stretched (see illustration below). Hold for a few seconds and return to your normal position. Repeat two or three times.

■ Exercise 7

Using a finger, apply pressure upwards from the eyebrow (see diagram below), holding the stretch for ten seconds.

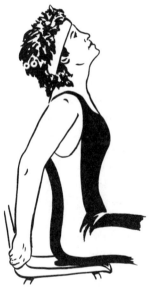

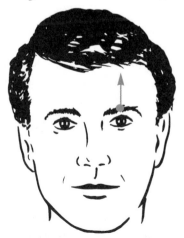

Pressure stretch from eyebrow

■ Exercise 8 *(over page)*

Far from having muscles in the neck and shoulders that are too rigid and 'tight', some people have neck and shoulder muscles that are too weak. The following exercise helps strengthen neck muscles: Clasp your hands together and place them on top of your head. Now press firmly downwards to contract the neck and tense the neck muscles. Hold this for ten seconds. Quickly remove your hands from the top of your head and gently stretch your neck upwards as in the diagram below.

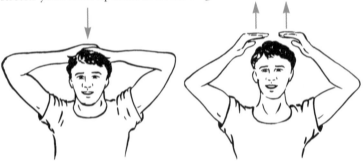

Stretching exercises for shoulders

Shoulders are not directly linked to the head and eyes but because they can affect neck muscles the following shoulder exercises may be helpful if your shoulders feel tense or stiff.

■ Exercise 1

If you are not warmed up it may be difficult reach the parts of your back you need to reach so start with the following routine: Breathing in, pull your shoulders up towards your ears. Breathe out, dropping your shoulders. Now breathe in and this time circle your shoulders in a forwards motion. Breathe out, circling your shoulders backwards and downwards.

■ Exercise 2

Standing or sitting (it doesn't matter which), bend your left arm above your head (see right) and bring your hand down to touch your right shoulder-blade (or as close as you can get). You should feel a stretch in the back of your upper arm. Repeat using your right arm to your left shoulder blade.

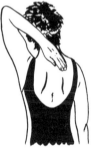

■ Exercise 3

Twist your right arm up behind your back and try to touch your left shoulder-blade. You should feel this stretch in your right shoulder. Repeat using your left arm.

■ Exercise 4

Now try combining exercises 2 and 3 so that you touch fingers behind your back, alternating arms. You'll probably find it is easier to do this one side than the other, and women usually find it easier than men. This is a difficult but excellent exercise for giving shoulders flexibility.

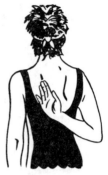

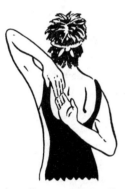

■ Exercise 5

Clasp your hands low down behind your back (see diagram right), elbows slightly bent. Holding your hands together tightly, pull down on your arms so that you feel a squeezing feeling between your shoulder blades. This will also produce a stretching feeling in your chest.

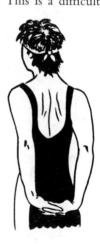

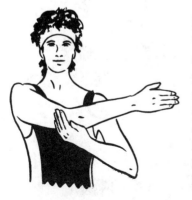

■ Exercise 6

With your left hand, pull your right arm firmly across in front of you, holding it just above the elbow. This will give you a feeling of stretch in your upper arm muscle and the back of your shoulder. Hold for a few seconds and let go. Repeat the exercise with your left hand pulling your right arm.

Using pressure points

Once you have softened and relaxed the neck muscles you can make use of certain 'pressure points' on the back of the neck to stimulate recovery even more.

This a special technique based on the ancient Chinese art of acupuncture, except that instead of using needles you use the pressure of your own (or a friend's) fingers. Another name for it is 'acupressure' and perhaps the best known form is the version developed many years ago in Japan called shiatsu.

As the diagram below shows, the area just under the skull is particularly important. Three main nerves – the major occipital nerve, the minor occipital nerve and the great auricular nerve – run through this area and pressure applied here can have enormous benefit to those with MS.

Apply finger pressure for about five or six seconds to each point and repeat the pressure up to eight times. The point may be tender at first but the tenderness will subside as the treatment progresses.

Having done the pressure points, massage around the whole area for about five minutes with firm sliding strokes of your hands, beginning at the nape of the neck and moving up to the skull. This is exactly the procedure that produced such excellent results when used on Connie (see 'Connie's story' on page 41).

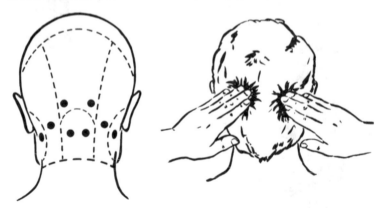

Pressure points on the neck for eye problems

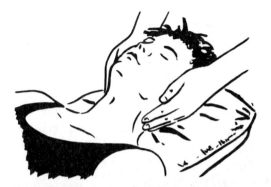

*Applying pressure
points on the neck
for eye problems*

Nutritional support

It is important, always, that any physical therapy is supported by the
right sort of nutritional therapy. That means by eating the right sort
of diet and, usually, supplementing that diet with extra vitamins,
minerals and amino acids. The question of diet is an important one
for me and I'll tell you why.

Like many people of my age I was not brought up to think too
much about what I ate or drank. We were the first of the hamburg-
ers and coke generation in Britain and that was what I had most of
the time for the first ten years of living with MS. No one, certainly
not the doctors, told me any different. But that was before I went
to the famous Peto Institute in Hungary.

In Hungary my diet changed dramatically – and not by choice
either. Hungary in those days was still under communism and that
meant food, as most other things, was in short supply. Shopping was
not so much a matter of going out with a list of what you wanted as
queuing up to see what you could get! Processed and prepackaged
food simply did not exist. And neither did cakes, pastries or sweets.
'Treats' for children in hungry Hungary in 1989 meant a piece of
badly bruised and discoloured fruit. In fact you could always tell when
bananas were in the shops by the length of the queues! Bananas were
as chocolate is to children in the west since there was no chocolate in
Hungary. But all this 'deprivation' had the most amazing effect on me.

After three weeks on pasta, vegetables, yoghurt, eggs, rice, fruit and
an occasional piece of chicken (if I was lucky!) I had lost all my excess

weight, my eyes sparkled, I had masses of energy and felt brilliant. It was a revelation. I realized then how much we have lost with our luxury lifestyles in the west and how much worse off we are health-wise. We have much to be grateful for too, of course, but healthy eating isn't one of them.

My experience in Hungary was a turning-point in my eating habits that continues to this day. And it also turned me on to the benefits to be had from taking supplements to support the low levels of nutrients in much modern factory-farmed foods. For eye problems the main supplements to note are vitamins A and B2.

■ Vitamin A *(preferably as beta carotene, its natural form)*

Vitamin A promotes the growth of healthy skin, hair, teeth and gums so it is a fundamental treatment for eye disorders. Specifically, experts know it helps in conditions of eye weakness, it counteracts night blindness and weak eyesight, and it aids in the treatment of many eye disorders.

The best natural sources of beta carotene are carrots, green and yellow vegetables, yellow fruits (melons and the like), eggs, milk and other dairy products, margarine, liver and fish liver oil.

Deficiency symptoms include mouth ulcers, poor night vision, acne, frequent colds and infections, dandruff, thrush, cystitis and diarrhoea. The recommended daily amount (RDA) is 7,500iu (international units) a day.

■ Vitamin B2 *(otherwise known as riboflavin)*

None of the B vitamins – there are about 17 so far discovered – are stored by the body and so they must be replaced regularly, either through the diet or by supplementation. A B-vitamin deficiency is the most common nutritional deficiency in America. Symptoms of deficiency are burning and itching sensations in the eyes, light sensitivity, dry lips.

Vitamin B2 promotes healthy skin, nails and hair, helps eliminate dry mouth, lips and tongue, benefits vision and eliminates eye fatigue. But all B vitamins are interdependent so, particularly in cases of stress such as happens in MS, a B-complex (a complex containing all B-vitamins in a well-balanced formula) should be taken.

The best natural food sources of vitamin B2 are milk, liver, kidney, yeast, cheese, green leafy vegetables, fish and eggs.

Reflexology

Reflexology, or reflex zone therapy as it also called, is a therapy based on the belief that the feet are a mini 'map' of the body and that various organs of the body are connected to specific areas or 'zones' on the feet (and also hands). The diagram below shows you the idea. The eyes and the neck are related to the big toe and the toe next to it, particularly to the base and sides of the toes.

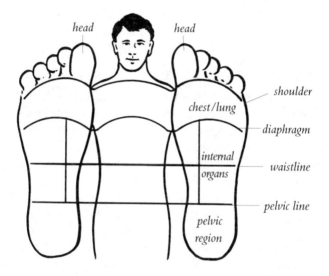

Reflexologists like myself believe that imbalances in the body can be detected by the sensitivity of the various parts of the feet and hands to pressure applied to them and that these imbalances can be put right by a particular sort of pressure or massage. (In reality the hands are usually only manipulated if it is too difficult to use the feet for any reason.)

There isn't a great deal of research for all this yet but there is little doubt reflexology benefits a large number of those who use it – so much so, in fact, that it is now being widely taken up by nurses and used in hospitals all over the world. In Britain it has even been recognised officially by the national Society of Physiotherapists.

In an ideal world we wouldn't have any need for reflexology because we would get all the therapy we need simply from walking around rough ground in bare feet. How lucky, in this respect at least, are those native people in parts of the world where they never wear shoes and socks! They have natural reflexology all the time – and certainly seem much healthier for it in many ways.

Of course we in the so-called 'civilised' west are used to wearing shoes these days and so reflexology, I feel, has become a 'must' that everyone, not just those with MS, should learn. This becomes especially pressing if you are someone who doesn't or can't walk or whose walking ability is limited, as indeed mine is. In these circumstances reflexology is a brilliant way of giving your whole internal system a good 'toning up'.

Reflexology and the central nervous system

According to reflexology, because the central nervous system links all parts of the body to every other part and passes signals to and fro between them, manipulation of those areas is said to directly affect and improve not only the function of that particular part of the nervous stem but the body as a whole.

As far as the head is concerned, the crucial area on the foot is the big toe. The rest of the nervous system – the spinal cord and the nerves that radiate out from it to the rest of the body – is represented by a line from the toe to the heel. Perhaps the most important reflex on the toe is that at the very top of the toe. This corresponds to the part of the brain known as the cerebral cortex. The cerebral cortex is our intelligence, the 'main brain' if you like, that controls everything from how we think, speak and learn to enjoying music and art.

Other important reflexes on the toe are those that relate to the glands of the endocrine system, the system that regulates the hormones that control everything from our appetite to our sexuality. The functions of the main endocrine glands are:

- the pineal gland (also known as the 'third eye') responds to light and plays a strong part in mood control
- the hypothalamus gland controls emotional response, appetite and body temperature
- the pituitary gland is the 'master gland', controlling the other glands
- the thyroid gland controls our metabolism which, in turn, affects energy levels
- the parathyroid gland affects calcium and phosphorus levels, both important for muscle tone and functioning.

The diagram on the below shows the parts of the toe that correspond to specific endocrine glands.

Perhaps the most important for people with MS are the pineal, the hypothalamus and the parathyroid. The parathyroid reflex point is often particularly sensitive in people with MS. The parathyroid is important not just because of its link to muscles but because it produces parathormone. Any drop in the level of this hormone can cause calcium levels in the blood to drop also, resulting in muscle-twitches, cramps and spasms common in MS.

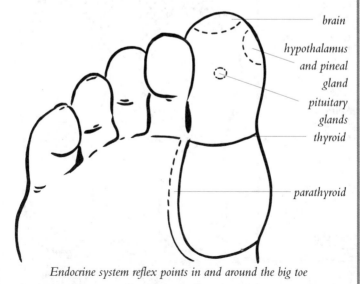

Endocrine system reflex points in and around the big toe

For neck and eye problems I gently massage the big toe and the toe next to it for two to three minutes. The reflex points for the eyes are on these toes (the right eye on the right toe and the left eye on the left toe, see the diagram below). Apply pressure up 'the back' of the second toe and to the base of all the toes. It may be tender at first but persevere. Things will improve.

Reflexology is a simple and perfectly safe technique that anyone can use. It can easily be learnt for self-help but it is much more effective if you can find someone, preferably a trained reflexologist, to do it to you (see 'Appendix C: Resources' for contact details).

If the person isn't a reflexologist ask them to support the foot in one hand and gently massage your toes with the other, particularly around the joint with the rest of the foot, and on the soft pad underneath. You may be surprised how good it feels and how much better you become in time.

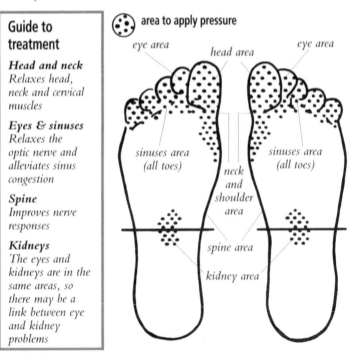

Guide to treatment

Head and neck
Relaxes head, neck and cervical muscles

Eyes & sinuses
Relaxes the optic nerve and alleviates sinus congestion

Spine
Improves nerve responses

Kidneys
The eyes and kidneys are in the same areas, so there may be a link between eye and kidney problems

area to apply pressure

eye area

head area

eye area

sinuses area (all toes)

neck and shoulder area

sinuses area (all toes)

spine area

kidney area

The reflexology points for eye problems

Patients' stories: *Leonie*

'I was diagnosed with MS at the end of 1988 at the age of 31 after having had trouble with my vision for about six months. The doctors had nothing to offer apart from a massive – and I mean massive – course of intravenous steroids that I didn't like and didn't seem to help. Then a nurse I spoke to recommended I see a homoeopath she knew.

'For four years I was treated by this very pleasant and competent man who gave me homoeopathic remedies to help my system detoxify itself, as he saw it, of whatever it was causing my symptoms.

'I don't know whether it was detoxification but what happened was that spots erupted all over my cheeks – and I don't mean the ones I sit on! In fact, I'd wake up every morning with an eruption. I complained endlessly but always got the same reply: 'Homoeopathy is not for the vain, and having spots is a good sign...'.

'I confess to being vain and so was horrified to see my once fine skin growing uglier, with pitted flesh and scarring, with almost every passing day. I'd laugh and joke about being the oldest adolescent with acne but inside it really hurt.

'Finally, in 1993, I was coerced by my family into stopping taking the remedies and going back, against my better judgement, to my doctor. He prescribed Dianette, a classic acne treatment for post-teenage women of oestrogen and anti-androgen tablets – but I wasn't prepared for what happened next.

'I'd only been taking the tablets for a couple of months when I was hit by a mass of weird, and frightening, symptoms. The double vision that had cleared with the homoeopathic remedies returned with a vengeance, and it was accompanied with mind-bending nystagmus – continuous rapid oscillation of the eyeballs.

'If you've ever had a television without vertical hold (and the desire to thump it on the top to rectify it!) you'll know exactly how I felt. But that was only the beginning.

'Slowly I lost all control over the muscles in my face. After a while my right eyeball wouldn't move. It remained static in its socket, staring eerily at people like a bloodshot glass eye, weeping involuntary tears because it couldn't even blink. Then, horror of horrors, my face started to distort. I looked like Quasimodo's apprentice as my nose, mouth and eyes all began twisting to the left.

'It was then my mother took me meekly back to the homoeopath, my face like an all-in wrestler, my eyes hidden behind sun-glasses. Within a week his remedies had straightened my face out. It took weeks to see properly but I persevered with his remedies, even though the spots returned. I considered it the lesser of the two evils.

'After a while, though, the double vision returned. I put it down to the stresses and strains of looking after two teenagers and a seven-year-old as well as having a husband whose job took him away from home for long spells. But this time, along with the usual attendant problems, I began losing the strength in my hands and legs. I resorted to having to crawl up stairs on my hands and knees and bump down again on my bottom!

'Finally, after I'd accidently smashed my favourite ornament, my sister-in-law suggested I try Susie's clinic-in-a-gym. It had been suggested many times before by many different people in Harwich, the Essex coastal town where we live and where everyone knows every-one else's business. Many different people had been effusive in their praise of the clinic – but I had remained sceptical.

'How could her gym help me? I asked them. I didn't have any mobility problems. All my troubles were in my eyes. But listening to my sister-in-law I decided to give Susie a try. Anyway I was desperate and I had nothing to lose.

'I started going to Under Pressure in 1994 and far from losing any-thing I have gained an awful lot. The gym-clinic uses gentle exercise combined with supervised breathing and dietary advice. It's a totally holistic approach to treatment that has helped me enormously. In fact I'm a million times better.

'I no longer have any weakness in my hands and legs and my eyes are completely better. In fact I am so symptom-free it is just as if I don't have MS and never did have.

'I'm enormously grateful to Susie and all her therapists for their intelligent, caring and, above all, positively cheerful approach to the treatment of MS.'

■ Comment

When Leonie first came to see me she told me she had had her tonsils removed when she was four because of recurring tonsillitis and had suffered as a child from bronchitis. She also had a bad fall from a horse in 1969, when she hurt her coccyx (her 'tail'), but did nothing about it even though it continued to hurt for many years afterwards.

In 1984 a bad 'flu virus laid her low and she found it very hard to shake it off. Around the same time she suffered a divorce, a death in the family and a miscarriage – all within a three-month period. Two years later she suffered a severe bout of bronchitis, resulting in her seriously neglecting her diet. The first symptoms of MS appeared soon after: sensitivity to the touch, as if something was crawling over her skin, and double vision in both eyes.

Because her problems were mostly upper body ones – Leonie had restricted movement in the neck and shoulders and upper thoracic muscle spasm as well as double vision – I concentrated my treatment on the neck and shoulder area. Her fatigue I treated with massage and diet.

A hair mineral analysis check – a special test to check the mineral content of the body using a sample of hair – showed that Leonie suffered from low blood sugar, a condition known as hypoglycaemia, and so she was also prescribed vitamin and mineral food supplements to help her.

Leonie improved quickly under the treatment. She has not relapsed and I now only ever see her for an occasional treatment when she feels like it.

Patients' stories: *Connie*

'I was 57 and enjoying yet another holiday in France with my husband in the autumn of 1987, taking a well-earned break from my job as a secretary with a firm of lawyers, when I felt pain in one of my legs. Back home in England I became aware that my eyesight was deteriorating, with periods of blurred vision.

'Visits to my optician and family doctor led to a referral to the famous Moorfields Eye Hospital in London, followed in April 1988 by three days in St Thomas's Hospital, also in London. The various tests and a lumbar puncture indicated MS – but neither my husband, a company secretary, nor I were told. My doctor simply told me I had neuritis of the eyes.

'It wasn't until October that I found out the truth when I read a magazine article about MS that mentioned the phrase 'demyelination'. It immediately struck a chord and I remembered I had seen it on one of my medical reports. When I asked my doctor outright whether he thought I had MS he admitted he did – but he said it was not normal medical practice to give such information to patients unless they demanded it.

'My initial reaction to the news of having this incurable disease was one of being deeply upset and, after the shock, some anger at not having been told at the outset. Conversations with other MS sufferers subsequently has revealed that this approach to patients on the part of doctors is far from uncommon. My husband and I told the doctor that we were both intelligent adults and deserved to be treated as such.

'After this confirmation we told everyone about my MS and family and friends offered huge and immediate help and support. None of it, however, quite compensated for the steady deterioration of my eyesight. This had become so bad that in February 1994 I was officially registered blind.

'Over the years my walking steadily worsened also and I began to need a walking stick or an arm to lean on to get about. Mentally I am alert as ever, which means frustration tended to creep in as I found I couldn't do the sort of simple tasks that used to be so easy. Into all this, in March 1992, came Susie and her clinic.

'My husband read about it in a local newspaper and since it was local we decided it might be worth trying. We both decided to go along – me for my MS and my husband to get his weight down! – and soon I was making twice weekly visits. When Susie and her devoted husband Ian opened their new purpose-built gym and clinic in February 1993 I was one of the first to make use of it.

'The difference all this made to my morale was enormous. Though physical benefit took some time to appear, the mental uplift of not being alone and working in a cheerful and bouyant atmosphere with other sufferers, some far worse off than I am, all showing such a positive spirit in spite of their condition, was wonderful.

'It made me realize that it is possible to remain optimistic in spite of MS and in spite of the fact I can no longer do many of the things I used to enjoy doing, such as driving, holidaying abroad, going to concerts and gardening. I can still listen to music and I enjoy 'talking books' and recreating the lost art of conversation!

'Recently, thanks to Susie, I have seen some physical improvement in my condition and that has helped me enormously. One of the therapists began massaging the muscles in my neck at the base of my skull and slowly but surely my eyesight has improved. At the time of writing it is perhaps 25 per cent better than it was.

'I had a regular checkup at Moorfields Hospital in August 1995 and they said there had indeed been a definite improvement. They even encouraged me to continue with the treatment since they said it appeared to be helping in a way they couldn't!

'I am naturally delighted and am sure it is down to Susie's treatment and the care and the insight of her staff. I am looking forward to further improvements – though I won't be too upset if they don't come. One of the important things Susie has taught me about MS is not to dwell on the things you can't do but concentrate on those things you can.

'MS constantly tries to dictate your life but however difficult it is it must not be allowed to – it must be firmly and resolutely pushed into the background. Above all, it is important to remain positive and never envy others. None of us knows what problems or traumas they may have hidden beneath their public face.

'I always hope for some remission and, in the long term, an eventual cure but I have already been luckier in my life than many people and I have much to be thankful for.'

■ Comment

From the moment Connie came to see me I felt sure there was something we could do to help. Her many symptoms other than eyesight problems and her long history of sinus problems and flu convinced me that there might be reasons for her condition other than MS.

When I examined her I found her back muscles were in total spasm – they were hard and inflexible – and she told me her neck and shoulders were painful when touched. This is the area we decided to concentrate on and the results are there for all to see. For Connie it was a case of literally seeing when she could not do so before treatment began.

Connie's eyesight has not returned completely and it is possible it may never do so. But at least she can now see enough to read the clock and recognize the faces of those around her. Best of all, Connie herself believes she will not now lose her sight completely — as doctors had told her she would — and so will be able to watch her beloved grandchildren grow up.

Connie is being encouraged to improve her previously poor diet and take extra vitamin and mineral supplements to help her condition even further and we will continue to treat her digestive and respiratory system as well as her back and shoulders. I am satisfied we have managed to stabilise her eyesight and my aim now is to see an improvement in her digestive and immune systems.

Who knows — we might do better yet. I hope so.

face, speech and balance

Symptoms of MS in the head, and particularly the face, are the familiar 'pins and needles' feeling, numb patches, pain (neuralgia), and paralysis. Obviously any of these can cause speech problems if the tongue and mouth area are affected. Anyone who's tried to speak after an injection at the dentist will know exactly how it feels.

Another common MS problem located mainly in the head – though it can have other origins – is loss of balance from infection in the inner ear or sinuses (see 'Balance problems in MS' on page 52).

Speech problems as the result of a face affected by MS are particularly unfortunate because they can make perfectly sensible, otherwise normal people sound drunk or stupid or both when, of course, they are neither.

My treatment for facial problems, including those affecting speech, are basically the same as treatment for the neck and eyes covered in the previous chapter. That is, massage and stretching exercises followed by application of the pressure points. Again, I find that reflexology can also be useful.

Massage for the face

Massage should concentrate on the strong rope-like muscle on either side of the neck (called the sternocleidomastoid muscle). Make sure you massage up the side of the face close by the ear and up to the temple area. This should be a light, gentle massage.

Another important area is that covered by the trigeminal nerve (see diagram on page 24). This is the largest cranial nerve and is responsible for the actions of both chewing and speech. It starts in the brain and spreads over the face in three branches:

- the opthalmic nerve (affecting the eyes)
- the maxillary nerve (affecting the lower jaw and cheekbone)
- the mandibular nerve (affecting the lower jaw only).

Again, MS-like symptoms can be displayed by people without MS because of a buildup of congestion in this area. This seems to be especially true, for example, of people with recurrent and persistent sinusitis. Congestion in the side of the face can affect speech and so give apparent symptoms of MS.

If you think this might apply to you, the following technique might help relieve the pressure: gently massage the area under the eyes and around the cheekbone and include a light tapping with the fingertips.

Stretching exercises for the face

Stretching the muscles of the body, not just of the face, is one of the most important exercises anyone with MS can do. Stretching is even more important than toning and strengthening. Stretching not only tones and strengthens muscles it extends them, keeping them supple, improving flexibility, mobility and circulation, and helping eliminate fatigue.

In fact, the benefits of stretching seem out of proportion for something so apparently simple and straightforward. But stretching is crucial for anyone, not just those with MS. When we get up in the morning and stretch and yawn without even thinking of it we are performing one of the most vital exercises of the day. Think of how a cat gets up a stretches and how supple they stay. Stretching 'wakes up' all our body systems, from our bones, muscles and sinews to our circulation, digestion and our hormonal (or endocrine) system.

So it is important to allow yourself time for a good stretch and yawn first thing in the morning. Yawning is the most basic of muscle stretching exercises for the face. But apart from yawning there are other exercises you can do that will have a very definite effect on specific areas of your face.

How stretching helps

Stretching areas on the face (and neck) stimulates glands that form part of the body's endocrine system to function better, especially the pituitary gland and the thyroid gland. The endocrine system is the system that controls the body's hormones, chemicals that control our most vital functions from our sexuality to how we digest food.

Carried in the bloodstream, hormones affect us in the most subtle of ways and it is the job of the various glands of the endocrine system to produce the right hormones at the right level. The pituitary gland, for example, controls the overall flow of hormones to make sure we have the right balance while the thyroid gland secretes the hormones that control our metabolism, the process by which what we eat and drink turns into cells in our body.

The pituitary gland, which is located in the centre of the brain, is stimulated by stretching the neck muscles and also by applying gentle pressure to the back of the neck high into the base of the skull (an area known as the medulla oblongata).

Light pressure in the areas to the right and left of the base of the neck helps the thyroid gland which is in the throat.

Stretching exercises in the mouth, jaw and neck areas also help the submaxillary and sublingual glands responsible for saliva and involved in the making and strengthening of bone tissue.

In general terms, stretching helps essential nutrients to reach the bones of the body via the spinal column, stimulates the blood supply to all parts of the body, and helps the digestive system by dispersing fats and toning internal organs and muscles. But take care to stretch at the right time. Stretching exercises should not be done:

- on an empty stomach (apart from an early morning stretch)
- when you are very weak or exhausted
- immediately after an accident
- if you have an injury or any internal inflammation.

For problems in the side of the face

For problems such as pain or numbness in the left hand side of the face, turn your head to the right and place the palm of the left hand in the nape of the neck, slightly to the left side, and the palm of the right hand on the right side of the forehead (see right). Now stretch upwards with the hands and hold this position for ten seconds. To treat the right of the face simply reverse the above positions. The benefit of this is accumulative, the more so if done in conjunction with other therapies.

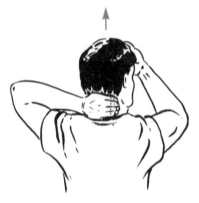

Pressure points for the face

In cases of numbness or pain, the application of pressure to the area of pain or numbness can be beneficial. Use the three middle fingers – the index, middle and third finger – and apply pressure for about 5–6 seconds to each area.

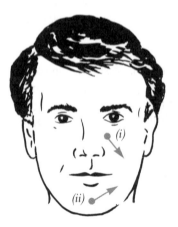

For problems in the upper jaw

Apply pressure with a finger or fingers below the eye in a downward direction, holding the stretch for ten seconds (see i left).

For problems in the lower jaw

Apply pressure on the chin in a diagonally upwards direction, holding the stretch for ten seconds (see ii left).

Reflexology for the face

The technique to be used is the same as that for the head and neck areas (see chapter 3). The important area where the face is

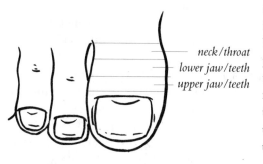

neck/throat
lower jaw/teeth
upper jaw/teeth

concerned is the front of the toe because this is the part that correponds to the face. The right toe corresponds to the right side of the face and the left toe to the left.

Manipulating this area can be beneficial for any problem to do with the face from neuralgia, toothache and skin problems to numbness, tingling and the loss of sensation.

Massaging the toes on each foot is also good for blocked sinuses (see diagram opposite). If you suffer from sinusitis (and sinusitis seems to be common among people with MS), or even if you used to but don't any longer, you may find that your toes are very tender to the touch. Persevere and the tenderness will wear off as your sinuses clear.

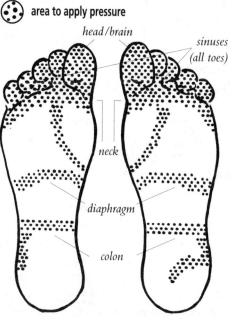

● area to apply pressure

head/brain

sinuses (all toes)

neck

diaphragm

colon

Reflexology points for sinusitis

Patient's story: **Liz**

'I was diagnosed with MS in 1985 when I was 29 after experiencing typical MS symptoms of altered feelings and numbness in various parts of my body, especially my face and hands.

'My face was particularly badly affected, with total numbness down the left side that affected my mouth, tongue and teeth and made me sound drunk when I tried to speak!

'In fact, though I can't pinpoint precisely the onset of my first symptoms, I can see looking back that I had probably begun the symptoms in my early twenties. I had a tendency to being clumsy and accident-prone. I would always be the one to knock over a glass of wine at a dinner party and crockery never lasted long in my flat! It was a bit of a joke with my friends and 'doing a Humphreys' (my maiden name) became a favourite saying of theirs whenever someone had a similar accident.

'My doctor suspected from the beginning that it was MS and kept referring me to the National Hospital for Neurological Diseases in London but it was 18 months before they confirmed MS. Previously they'd always said it was stress. But eventually an MRI scan showed the tell-tale lesions in my brain.

'When the doctors finally came out with it I was devastated and the initial shock of it resulted in what I can only describe as my first major relapse.

'My feelings about my situation were governed by the fact that someone I knew with MS was in a wheelchair. But shock quickly gave way to a determination to fight back – especially after meeting two people, fellow sufferers, who did more than anyone else to show me how it is possible to rule MS rather than let it rule you.

'The first of these was a young woman, a few years younger than me, I met when I was undergoing tests at the National Hospital. She was recovering from a relapse that had left her totally paralysed and was a shining example of the power of a positive spirit. She was a tremendous source of encouragement, information, help and support and remains a good friend to this day.

'The second person was Susie Cornell. I met Susie just before

Christmas in 1992 when a friend, another MS sufferer, wanted me to benefit from the same programme that had helped her. I have been attending Susie's pioneer centre in Chelmsford for two-and-a-half years now and I must say it has been a revelation.

'Before I went I had this numbness in my face, just like I'd had an injection from the dentist, but now I am completely free of the numbness. I must say it does tend to return in times of stress but Susie and her team give me neck massage and reflexology and that takes it away again very quickly afterwards, usually in two days.

'What I particularly like is that Susie has always encouraged me in all the areas I have investigated in my determination that I was not going to end up in a wheelchair.

'For example, I had very quickly decided that diet played a significant part in MS and since my existing diet was pretty poor I had worked very hard on making changes, including taking supplements such as evening primrose oil. Susie supported me in all this and many other things besides.

'A hair analysis showed I was high in a lot of toxic metals like aluminium and she was able to advise me on what supplements to take to help detoxify my body and correct its chemical balance.

'One day I came to her centre after a particularly stressful time at home only able to walk with the help of a stick. It was the only time I can remember ever having had a problem with walking and everyone was most concerned. But after just one session on what Susie calls her "nerve gym" equipment I got up and walked away quite normally. I'd forgotten I had a problem at all!

'I have always believed that self-help is the key to success and Susie's programme is geared very much to encouraging individuals to do just that. My MS is of the relapsing-remitting kind but everyone is different and over the years I have tried hard to find the right combination of treatments that work for me.

'When I was first diagnosed I tried hyperbaric oxygen but I'm not sure this helped. On the other hand I think the better diet and the food supplements definitely have. So has Susie's programme.

'I always used to feel tired and was often irritable, especially since I now have a husband and two young children, aged 6 and 4. But I see all these things in a positive light. I still have symptoms of MS but the tiredness and irritability have gone and the children's understanding of "Mummy's wibbly-wobbly legs" will also increase as they get older.

'One unexpected benefit of the supplements is that my PMS also seems to have gone.

'Whilst I am always aware of my many and varied symptoms, and have to adapt my life accordingly, these days I am able to function reasonably well thanks to the treatments I am getting and give myself.

'I still get relapses about every two years or so – when I'm severely incapacitated for several weeks – but I know that I can help myself get better quicker by maintaining a positive attitude and that is the most valuable thing anyone with MS can learn.' [September 1995]

■ Comment

When Liz came to see me she was still suffering from the whiplash effects of a car accident in 1990 that had left her with severe restriction of her neck muscles and upper thoracic area. In addition she told me she had very bad growing pains as a child, with a number of throat infections and tonsillitis.

At the time she first started experiencing symptoms of MS, around 1979, she had just recovered from a very bad bout of 'flu, which she had taken a long time to shake off and a series of emotional traumas and an erratic lifestyle had meant she had seriously neglected her diet..

A few years earlier she had had a bad car accident, when her car had hit a brick wall, leaving her very bruised and shaken, and a few years before that she had had a major back operation that had put her in hospital for two months. While she was in hospital her mother had died.

We gave Liz physical therapy for the restricted movement in her upper body and neck, reflexology, a dietary 'detoxification' programme and food supplements.

The physical therapy consisted of ultrasound, faradism and manipulation, all of which helped. More dramatic, though, was that after only three sessions of reflexology Liz found her face had lost its numbness and returned to normal.

A hair analysis showed that Liz suffered from an excess of aluminium and copper and so was put on a special dietary programme to eliminate their effects. This was reinforced later with nutritional supplements.

Balance problems in MS

A number of people with MS suffer from loss of balance. The cause can be problems in the head with the inner ear and sinuses but other causes can be low blood pressure, low blood sugar *(hypoglycaemia)*, malnutrition/maldigestion and breathing incorrectly (see page 68).

Whatever the cause I advise anyone with persistent balance problems to see a doctor for a medical check. Even if the reason is just a minor ear or sinus infection it is best to make sure it is only that and not something more serious. Having established that it is nothing serious you can start to do something about it.

Sinus problems, including infection of the sinuses *(sinusitis)*, are common in people with MS who also seem to have a tendency to suffer from catarrh. To me this suggests, again, some weakness in the immune system and so treatment needs to address this basic problem rather than just go out and buy some nasal spray over the counter. A spray may give temporary relief but will do nothing to remove the root cause of the catarrh – and in fact will usually make it worse in the long-term.

Treatment for sinusitis and catarrh

Treatment for catarrh and sinusitis includes changing diet, nutritional support with food supplements, and reflexology.

■ Diet

The most important thing is to limit dairy products, especially milk and cheese. Cow's milk is a known cause of catarrh as well as allergies.

■ Nutritional support

The nutrients most effective are vitamin A, vitamin C, and zinc.

Vitamin A *(preferably as beta carotene)*

Vitamin A protects and strengthens the mucous membranes lining the nose, throat and lungs but a deficiency can allow harmful bacteria a home in which to 'lodge'. That's a major reason why many people with MS seem unable to throw off colds and catarrh, especially in the winter months and more especially if they have resorted to standard over-the-counter drug treatments. Many of the ingredients in such cold remedies actually lower the levels of vitamin A in the blood – and so, far from improving things, they actually make the situation worse!

The moral here is obviously if you ever get a cold or inflammed nose, sinuses, throat or lungs try natural remedies before any of the heavily advertised brands at your local pharmacist.

The right dose of beta carotene (natural viamin A) is 7,500iu a day. Never exceed this dose if you are pregnant or planning to be so: Vital though vitamin A is, too much can cause brain damage to the unborn child.

Vitamin C

Take 1-2 grams a day – but stop or cut down if you get diarrhoea. Remember, vitamin C is nothing like as effective on its own as when it is taken together with zinc. Zinc, a mineral, works to 'release' the full potential of vitamin C.

Zinc

Take 15mg of zinc (with vitamin C of course!). Zinc for colds and sinusitis is best taken as a lozenge you suck or chew.

Note Aspirin and corticosteroids (such as cortisone and prednisone, commonly used for arthritic pain, for example) can lower levels of vitamin C and zinc in the body. So doses may need to be higher if you are routinely taking either of these drugs.

■ Reflexology

The reflexes to treat are shown on page 49.

Balance problems caused by vitamin and mineral deficiency

The nutrient well known to affect balance if there is not enough of it in the body is vitamin B12 (see box on the following page: 'The importance of vitamin B12 in MS'), but another is the mineral manganese.

Manganese

Manganese deficiency can lead to dizziness and balance problems by causing imbalances in the middle ear. Good food sources are green leafy vegetables, peas and whole grain cereals. Manganese is also in tea (a cup contains about one milligram). But manganese can also be readily taken as a food supplement. The recommended daily dose is 5–25mg.

Vitamin B12

Vitamin B12 is only found in animal-based foods. Good sources are liver, beef, kidneys, eggs, milk and cheese. This important vitamin is often deficient in people with MS as it is in vegans (and so a vegan with MS is particularly at risk). Taking B12 as a supplement is one solution. The right dose is 100mcg a day – although any B vitamin should only be taken as a complex: that is, with all B vitamins together in one capsule. But for the reasons explained in the box below B12 is often given by injection to people with MS.

The importance of vitamin B12 in MS

Vitamin B12 is one of the most important nutrients in MS because B12 is vital to the healthy growth and repair of nerves. Severe B12 deficiency can cause permanent damage to the nervous system. Symptoms of B12 deficiency can take up to five years to show after the body's reserves have been used up.

Symptoms of B12 deficiency are tingling or numbness in the hands and feet, pain the ends of the fingers and toes, problems with balance, memory and concentration, mental confusion and depression, exhaustion, shortness of breath, problems with mucuous membranes, and anaemia. (Anaemia is caused by iron deficiency but because B12 helps to 'release' iron a B12 deficiency may be the real underlying reason.)

Other people likely to be B12 deficient are those from a family with an inherited tendency to pernicious anaemia, and those from families in which blue eyes and premature greying are common.

Certain drugs can also affect levels of B12 in the body. For example, prolonged use of antibiotics such as neomycin, some anti-diabetic drugs, the cholesterol-lowering agent cholestyromine, and potassium chloride supplements can all reduce levels of B12 and create a deficiency.

The trouble with B12 if you have MS, though, is that it is not really enough to take a capsule or the right food. According to my research *(see Appendix B)*, one of the features of MS is a lack of the right digestive enzymes and so people with MS often have difficulty absorbing B12 in the normal way through the stomach wall. That's why B12 is usually given to people with MS by injection: the stomach is by-passed and the vitamin goes straight into the blood supply where it is needed. Injection is normally done by a medical doctor.

More information on how to take supplements properly and effectively (and when not to take them) is in Appendix C.

hands
and arms

Lack of control over the movement and coordination of your hands and arms, such as dropping things, being generally clumsy and not being able to keep your hands steady, are classic MS symptoms. They may be accompanied by the usual pins-and-needles, and a variety of aches and pains from a severe burning feeling, as if you were on fire, and shooting pains to more general throbbing and tingling.

Another, less well-known, symptom is a heightened sensitivity to touch in specific areas of skin , seemingly unconnected to any other area. But again, and as I've already stressed, these symptoms can also be caused by problems that have nothing to do with MS.

The reason for this is the way the bones, muscles, tissues (our *musculoskeletal system,* see next page) and nerves of the body connect up and work.

As already explained in Chapter 2, everything in the body is connected to and runs through the back bone and spinal cord. The spinal cord is the body's principal nerve, a sort of 'mains cable' that runs through the middle of the back bone (in fact not one but many bones that make up what is known as the *vertebral column)* and sends out a network of nerves to every organ and fibre in your body.

The spinal cord is a part of the brain – it is literally an extension of it – and it acts as the central communications channel for the whole body. Messages and signals pass back and forth through it all the time,

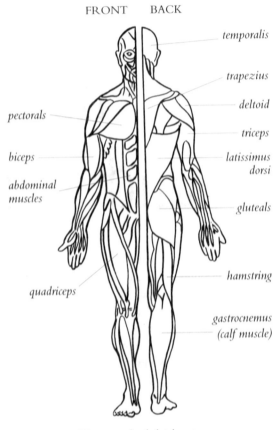

FRONT   BACK

temporalis

trapezius

deltoid

triceps

pectorals

latissimus
dorsi

biceps

abdominal
muscles

gluteals

hamstring

quadriceps

gastrocnemus
(calf muscle)

The musculo-skeletal system

linking the brain to the furthest limbs.

The back bone is basically the structure that keeps us upright and prevents everything collapsing in an untidy heap on the floor. But the backbone is held in place and is moved by quite strong broad bands of muscle that cover our backs. These same muscles also help support our heads and necks and affect our arms.

Looked at from the rear, muscles on our back run from below the shoulder diagonally to the waist – giving the familiar triangular shape to the upper part of the body – and these are supported by other groups of muscles around the shoulders and hips. Together these large muscles facilitate the complex movements of our arms and legs. Because of the way they are all interconnected and overlap, problems felt in the neck and shoulders may have their source lower down and vice versa.

As far as the hands and arms are concerned the vital muscles are in the upper area of the back known as the upper thoracic area. The rhomboid muscles between the shoulder blades and the spine are particularly important. Problems with the hands are often simply the result of tight cervical muscles and 'knotted' rhomboid muscles.

Not very long ago, for example, I had a problem with the middle finger of my left hand. It was slower to respond than the other fingers and was not picking up as quickly. Gently 'palpating' or feeling around my back, one of my therapists found that the rhomboid muscle on the left of my spine was very tender to the touch. It felt 'knotted', like a small piece of gristle. Light massage, becoming firmer as the tenderness subsided, coupled with acupressure, removed the problem after just three sessions (each session lasting about ten minutes). Stretching the muscles after the massage also helped the treatment to be quicker and more effective.

A longer-standing problem – known medically as a 'chronic' problem – is likely to take longer to clear but will also respond well to this sort of approach if it is done properly and with care.

A variety of treatments can help many of the problems of hands and arms caused by MS and, again, they consist broadly of massage, exercises, nutritional support and reflexology. Breathing exercises also help. Massage, stretching and exercise are particularly important to keep hands and arms strong and flexible.

Massage

A general massage to the upper neck area as described in chapter 3 and the upper rhomboids (between shoulder blades and spine), especially the area between the shoulder and collarbone, will help both hands and arms as well as the body as a whole. The upper chest area holds both the main lymph nodes or 'glands' that form a major part of the body's immune system (the nodes are actually in the front of the chest). Waste matter or 'toxins' damaging to the body collect in these nodes and so massaging gently in this area for perhaps ten minutes or so helps the fluid in the lymph system to work the collected material out of the nodes and so be eliminated by the body. A 'cleaner' lymph system means a healthier body.

Massage for hands and arms

The diagram below shows the area of the important rhomboid or 'shoulder-blade' muscle. The massage should be done using the thumb, strengthened if necessary by the other hand, to make deep stroking movements. In the case of the rhomboid muscle, work across the muscle from the outside of the shoulder towards the spine in the direction shown by the arrows in the diagram. Any bumps or lumps felt need to have extra pressure applied until they disappear. This may cause some discomfort, which may include tingling down the arm and into the fingertips as well as at the site of the lump itself, and it may

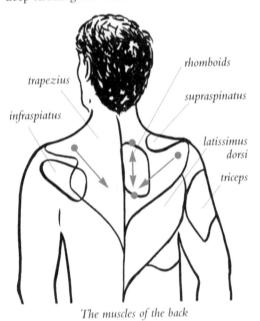

The muscles of the back

need more than one massage to work but persevere. It will be worth it.

Massage for hands

To massage your hands, apply hand cream or massage oil to both hands and rub them together. Make circles with your wrists in both directions, clockwise and anti-clockwise. This will warm them up ready for the following routine:

- Hold each finger in turn between your thumb and forefinger (of the opposite hand, obviously!) and gently press along its sides, back and front surfaces, working from the joint to the tip. Do the same with the thumb.

● Hold each finger in turn, again between finger and thumb, and gently pull and twist it. Repeat the procedures for both hands, including the thumbs.

● Make a fist with your hands and then stretch and spread your fingers and thumbs and imagine you are playing on a piano.

● Find a hard surface and make small tapping movements on it for a good couple of minutes so you feel the vibration going up your arm.

● Using your thumb, massage the whole of the palm of each hand in turn. The same reflex points that exist in the feet exist in the hands so massaging your palms can have the same benefits as reflexology. Make creeping movements with your thumbs, working into the web of the palm upwards towards your fingers.

● Finish by massaging up your hands towards your wrists with stroking movements, and continue up over your wrists onto your forearms.

When NOT to massage

Massage is generally a very safe and effective therapy but there are some situations in which it is inadvisable and can even be dangerous. Do not use massage in any of the following situations:

■ in cases of fever
■ over varicose veins
■ over recent scar tissue
■ over any septic areas (boils, spots etc)
■ over any pain of unknown cause or swelling
■ over broken skin, cuts or skin conditions such as eczema or psoriasis
■ during pregnancy, especially over the abdomen
■ in cases of severe heart conditions or 'weak' heart
■ in cases of very high or low blood pressure
■ in cases of diabetes
■ epilepsy
■ during an asthmatic attack
■ if in any doubt you are doing the right thing

Stretching exercise for hands

Place the tips of the fingers and thumb of both hands firmly together as in the illustration right and press so that the fingers spread out and the little fingers make a line horizontal with the floor. But it is important that the fingers don't actually meet, only the tips of each finger should touch. Hold the stretch for ten seconds and release. Repeat three times, pausing for a few seconds between each stretch.

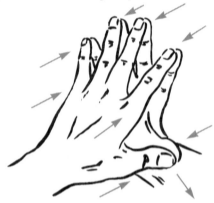

■ Massage for arms

This can be done by yourself or, better, by a friend. As with the fingers, massage cream or oil over the whole of the arm first. This will help to warm the arm up ready for the treatment. Then proceed as follows:

● Start by making long, sweeping movements up the inside of one arm and down the outside of it, increasing the pressure as you go. Do this four or five times.

● Holding the forearm firmly, make kneading and twisting movements with its muscles, again increasing pressure as you go and working in deeply with the thumb. Work into the spaces between the muscles and bones. Do the same with the upper arm but with less pressure, squeezing rather than digging into the muscles. Repeat the process on the other arm.

● Finish with long sweeping movements over the whole of each arm in turn.

Note MS makes the arms of some people extremely tender to the touch so start very gently, increasing the pressure only very gradually over time as tolerance builds up, as it will.

Stretching exercises for arms

● Extend one arm with the palm up. Gripping the wrist with the other hand, thumb down, gently but firmly pull the arm out and down. The arm being held should feel stretched. Hold the stretch for ten seconds and then release slowly and relax. Repeat the exercise three or four times. Do the same with the other arm.

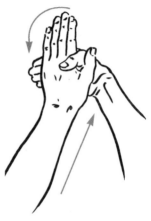

● Again, extend one arm but this time with the palm down. With the other hand, hold the extended hand with the thumb up around the base of the fingers and the other fingers around the hand (see illustration right). Now bend the fingers on the first hand backwards and hold for ten seconds. Repeat three or four times. Do the same on the other arm.

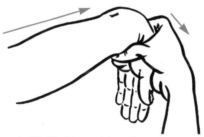

● To stretch the fore-arm, extend one arm with the palm again down and with the other hand bend the fingers down towards the fore-arm (see illustration above). Hold this position for ten seconds and release. Repeat three our four times as before. Do the same with the other arm.

● Finally, extend both arms out in front of you with palms facing out and fingers interlocked (see diagram right). Stretch upwards and away from you and hold for ten seconds. Repeat three to four times, releasing and relaxing briefly between each stretch.

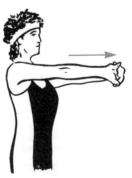

Exercises

A variety of hand–eye coordination and arm mobility exercises created originally at the famous Peto Institute in Hungary have been developed by me especially for MS and over the years many people have been kind enough to say they have found them immensely useful.

Simplicity is the key to these exercises that range from finger-tapping to arm-raising. Follow the sequence below for best results. The following exercises are also on my video *MS - A Home Video Programme* and in Appendix A 'Exercises for the arms' on page 162. (Appendix A also includes information on how to get a copy of the video).

■ Exercise 1

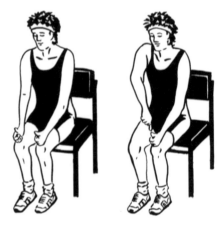

Sit squarely on a chair without arms and with both feet on the ground. Place your clenched fists on your knees with the thumbs pointing up. Swing one arm round behind you in a circular motion, like doing the 'front crawl' in swimming, and bring the thumb down to join the thumb on the opposite knee. Do the exercise slowly and deliberately to a count of five and try and keep your arms as straight as possible. To the same count, reverse the action so your fist with the thumb still sticking up returns to its original knee. Repeat the exercise using each finger of the same hand in turn. Now do the same thing with the other arm.

■ Exercise 2

Sit in the same way as in the previous exercise. Lift one fist up to touch your chin with the raised thumb. Repeat the action, this time touching the end of your nose with your thumb. Next, raise your

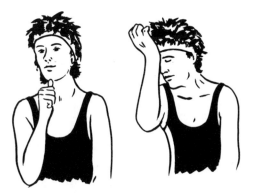

hand and touch your forehead with the inside of the wrist before returning your hand to your knee with the thumb still pointing up. Do the same thing with each of the other fingers of the same hand in turn. Now repeat the exercise with the other hand. Finally, do the whole exercise again with your eyes closed.

■ Exercise 3

Remain sitting on the chair but for this exercise you'll need a thin stick or knitting needle. Place the stick or needle on the floor just in front of your feet. Keeping your arms straight and using your thumb and index finger bend down and pick up the stick with both hands. Do this to the count of five. Holding the stick only between

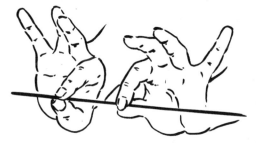

the thumb and one finger, change the fingers holding the stick starting with the index finger and moving through to the little finger and back again – a bit like playing the piano. Do this five times. Now repeat the exercise using just one hand, then the other, and finally both hands together again. Try doing it with your eyes closed. It's not easy but this exercise is one of the very best for improving coordination so persevere. It does get easier!

■ Exercise 4

You'll need a helper for this one. Sit in a sturdy chair with your helper standing behind you and his or her hands on your shoulders. Holding tightly onto your knees ask your helper to pull you gently back into an upright position while you resist as hard as you can. Allow your feet to come off the ground if necessary but pull yourself forward keeping hold of your knees and your head down. Keep up the pressure for a full five seconds. Repeat five times. Now do the exercise without holding your knees and your arms out straight in front of you as in the diagram opposite. As

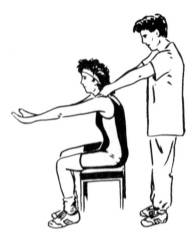

you get stronger ask your helper to increase the resistance so you have to work even harder.

■ Exercise 5

Still sitting on the chair, hold your arms out to the side with the hands cocked up and palms facing out. Making small circles, move your

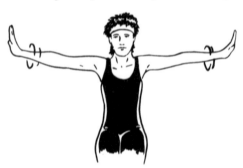

arms ten times forwards and then ten times backwards. Repeat the exercise using first one arm only and then the other. See left.

■ Exercise 6

On the same chair, sit upright with your back straight and your knees and feet slightly apart. Holding one arm verti-cal, pointing at the ceiling, make ten large forward circular move-ments. Repeat using the other arm. Now do the same thing again with both arms at once. See diagrams at the top of the next page.

My tip for strengthening hands and wrists: Carry around a tennis ball or soft sponge-ball and squeeze it as many times as possible throughout the day.

Exercise 6

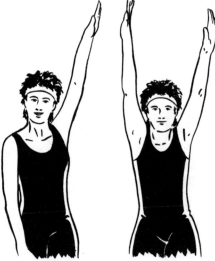

Exercises for those in wheelchairs

The following two exercises will help those in wheelchairs to exercise their shoulders and arms most effectively. They are done using 'stretch bands', large rubber bands readily available from sports and fitness centres especially for exercising in this way. They are best used with the help of someone assisting but you can do the following exercises just as well on your own by using chairs or door handles to anchor the 'spare' end.

▓ Arm lifts

Secure one end of the stretch band by looping it under the seat or armrest of the chair. Loop the other end around your upper arm as in the diagram on the following page. Now keeping firmly seated move your arm up and down, stretching the band as much as you can. Try and aim to bring your arm up to the horizontal position against the pull of the band. Do this five times. Repeat with the other arm. This exercise is particularly good for the shoulder muscles and you'll probably feel them protest at first but persevere.

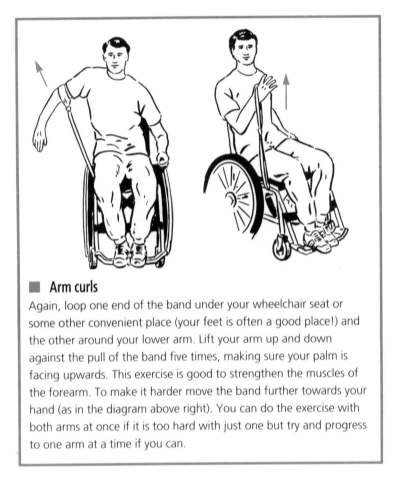

■ Arm curls

Again, loop one end of the band under your wheelchair seat or some other convenient place (your feet is often a good place!) and the other around your lower arm. Lift your arm up and down against the pull of the band five times, making sure your palm is facing upwards. This exercise is good to strengthen the muscles of the forearm. To make it harder move the band further towards your hand (as in the diagram above right). You can do the exercise with both arms at once if it is too hard with just one but try and progress to one arm at a time if you can.

Nutritional support

As with the head and neck, the B vitamins are of most help in problems with hands and arms – as they are for the body as a whole. Because B vitamins work together, and so should not be taken in isolation from each other, take a good quality B-complex for best results. The recommended daily dose is 50mg. Good natural sources of B vitamins are brewer's yeast, molasses, avocados, bananas and wheatgerm/oatgerm.

Reflexology

As described in earlier chapters, reflexology has a great deal to offer in the treatment of MS in my experience. For hands and arms the area on the foot to treat is the outside edge of the foot from the little toe down to about a third of the way along (see diagram below). Also important are the toes themselves, particularly those that relate to the base of the neck and the area on the spine known as the seventh cervical vertebra.

As before, the way of treating is to apply gentle pressure with fingers or thumb for a few seconds. There may be some tenderness and pain at first but as it subsides increase the pressure. Someone in a weakened state will be more sensitive than others so be sure to be particularly careful if you are trying to help someone in this condition.

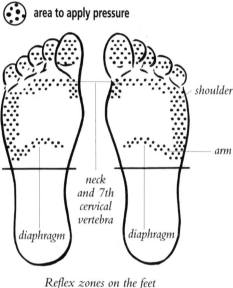

area to apply pressure

shoulder

arm

neck and 7th cervical vertebra

diaphragm   diaphragm

Reflex zones on the feet

Breathing exercises

Proper breathing is important for anyone, not just those with MS, because breathing is how we get oxygen into our bloodstream – and without oxygen nothing in our body works! People with MS tend to be shallow breathers – that is, they don't get enough good, fresh oxygen into their lungs – and that means harmful toxins stay in the body and don't get moved on and out as they should. This, in turn, affects the function of muscles and nerves and allows the buildup of painful toxins in the joints.

The key to correct breathing is to get your diaphragm, the large dome of muscle that sits under your lungs, to do the job it is supposed to do – pushing up on your lungs to empty and fill them properly. This is known as 'abdominal breathing' and is far better and healthier for you than breathing with your chest, known as 'thoracic breathing' (see the diagram below).

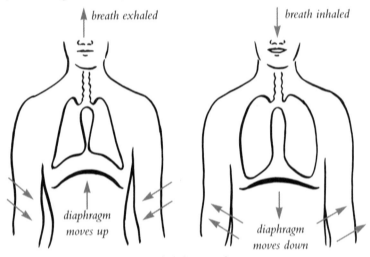

How to breathe correctly

The following breathing exercises should be done three times a day, preferably before you get out of bed in the morning and when you go to bed last thing at night as well as at regular intervals throughout the day:

Exercise for the lungs

- lie flat on your back on your bed
- bend your knees up so that your back and feet are flat on the bed
- relax all your muscles as much as you can (it sometimes helps to have your eyes closed for this)
- place one hand on your stomach
- breathe in to a count of one and out to a count of one
- breathe in to a count of two and out to a count of two
- continue breathing in and out to longer and longer counts, up to seven or eight.

Exercise for the diaphragm

- lie flat on your back (or stand up straight, it doesn't matter as long as your back is straight)
- slowly take a deep breathe in, filling your lungs as much as you can
- tighten your stomach muscles, pulling them as flat as possible
- still holding your stomach muscles, breathe out so you empty your lungs as completely as possible
- hold that position for one second and then release
- repeat the whole exercise for about five minutes and then relax.

Deep breathing exercise for the daytime

The following exercise is also for the diaphragm and is excellent for reducing stress as well as improving breathing. It can be done anywhere.

- Sit comfortably somewhere with your back straight. It can be on a chair or cross-legged on a cushion on the floor. Or you can lie on the floor if you prefer. The important thing, as with all the exercises, is to keep your back straight.
- Uncross your legs and arms and relax.
- Use your imagination now to see your lungs as two vast containers and your diaphragm under them as the bottom of these containers and made of rubber. Under the diaphragm, below your belly-button, imagine a magnet that will attract rubber.
- Breathe in and as you breathe in imagine the magnet is attracting your diaphragm towards it, allowing your lungs to expand to their maximum and fill completely with good, clean air.
- Now imagine the magnet shuts off, relaxing your stomach and allowing your diaphragm to spring back and push air out of your lungs. You are breathing out. Imagine your diaphragm is pushing all the air out of your lungs this way.
- Breathe like this for five minutes, concentrating on breathing with your stomach rather than your chest and shoulders and allowing your breathing to be as unforced and natural as possible, as if someone was doing it for you rather than you 'making' it happen.

Reflexology for better breathing

Start by stimulating the respiratory system (the lungs and diaphragm) by working on the reflexology points shown on the next page. The area on the balls of the feet relates to the lungs, the base of the big toe to the throat, the other toes to the sinuses and across the foot about half way down to the diaphragm. Work on these areas will help the respiratory system to work better and so make better use of the breathing exercises on pages 68–70.

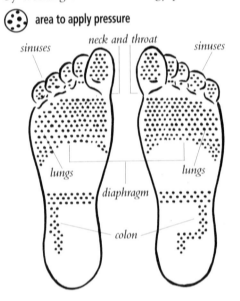

Respiratory reflex points

Special note about exercise and MS

Exercise has a very important part to play in the daily life of anyone with MS. Exercise not only helps to maintain function but prevent complications that can also result from inactivity such as bladder infection. The best sort of exercise programme is one that combines flexibility with strength and aerobic conditioning or stamina.

In MS maintaining muscle flexibility through stretching is perhaps the most important routine of all. Stretching prevents muscles contracting and contorting. But building up muscle strength and over-all stamina are important too if you want to stop an MS problem becoming a wider and more serious problem. It is very easy for disability to become anything from heart disease and hypertension (high blood pressure) to diabetes, arthritis and osteoporosis if you do not do all in your power to keep fit and healthy.

Keeping fit has positive benefits, too, of course. It will not only increase your physical independence (easing any burden you may feel on those nearest and dearest to you and making it easier for you to join in family and social activities) but improve your image of yourself and reduce any depression you may feel.

At this point, though, I must bring in an important caution. In MS, unlike in many other conditions, the exercise you do must be the right sort of exercise for you. Too much exercise or the wrong sort of exercise can do more harm than good, resulting in extreme tiredness and fatigue. I have had direct experience of this myself in the days when I was first finding out about 'alternative' treatments for MS.

Exercise only made me feel worse but I discovered this was because I was doing the wrong sort of exercise. I made this discovery when I visited the Peto Institute in Hungary in 1988. Although I went there with high hopes I very soon found myself almost rebelling against what they were doing with me. All I was getting out of it was fatigue!

The first thing they made me do was lie on a very uncomfortable wooden slatted bed. Turning onto to my left side – my weak side – to exercise was so painful they had to put special padding between me and the bed because I couldn't take the pain. Everything was so exhausting I had to stop every couple of minutes to rest.

The exercise class at the institute lasted about 45 minutes and I can honestly say I hated every minute of it at first and couldn't wait for it to be over. The trainers – they call them 'conductors' – were wonderful and always seemed to know exactly when I had had enough. But though they understood completely how I felt they would not let me give up. And I'm glad now they wouldn't.

I was at the Peto for three weeks on that first visit. Every day Monday to Friday for about an hour I went through their routine – and at the end I was transformed. Before I arrived I could not climb up or down stairs but after the treatment I was doing both, slowly perhaps but I was doing it. I had also dispensed with the padding on the wooden bed.

In fact it was not until I returned home to England that I realized how much benefit I'd had. I was no longer exhausted by the smallest

The role of exercise

Compared with our ancestors, the lives of most people today are devoid of what I call naturally-occuring exercise. That is, until quite recent times the majority of the population of the world exercised muscles and limbs quite adequately as a natural and normal part of the daily struggle to survive: pushing, pulling, lifting, carrying, walking and running. Today, though, thanks to modern technology and labour-saving gadgetry, most people, particularly in the western world, no longer work their muscles as they did – and should.

Even our inbuilt 'fight or flight' responses are not used in the way they were developed in us to be used. These days it is threatening letters from the bank that get our adrenalin running rather than escape from a sabre-toothed tiger!

Without exercise, our muscles lose their elasticity and our joints their flexibility, artery walls harden and blood vessels clog up, the immune system doesn't work as well and we get more problems with our digestive system. The result is we get older quicker and iller sooner than we should. Lack of exercise can be responsible for a wide range of problems such as poor circulation, high blood pressure, heart disease, rheumatism, arthritis, stress diseases, diabetes, and even – perhaps ironically – tiredness and fatigue.

Regular exercise raises the body's metabolic rate and keeps it raised for up to 48 hours. This increase in the rate copes naturally and correctly with all manner of factors in most people's daily lives such as the famous, and potentially deadly, 'fight or flight' stress responses. So you can see that the best way to cope with most of the so-called 'diseases of ageing' such as stiffness, aching joints, overweight, tiredness, and being constantly ill is to exercise regularly. That means ideally every two or three days at least. But the right sort of exercise is also important.

The right sort of exercise is not 'pumping iron' to build muscles or fast-moving aerobics but exercise that mimics basically the 'resistance' exercises of everyday living as it used to be (pushing, pulling, lifting, carrying and so on). I have found that resistance exercising – which is the basis of all the exercises I offer at 'Under Pressure' – is the best form of exercise for strengthening the immune system.

task and had enjoyed the exercises so much I actually missed doing them.

The Peto exercises are now part of my everyday life. They are so simple and easy anyone can do them at any time of the day, standing at the sink or sitting in a chair. You don't have to make time for them. They can fit into any routine and become as normal as breathing. I have got into the habit of regularly doing calf muscle lifts and stretches as I do the washing-up for example. These are the exercises I have now put on video for anyone to benefit from – and many of them are in this book.

I said earlier it is important to try and remain as active as possible but it is just as important in MS to exercise with care. At the Peto Institute I was being pushed with care by people who knew exactly what they were doing. People with MS without the same level of expert care should exercise with caution. In particular:

- Do not over exercise. Over exercising can harm otherwise healthy muscles. Limit your time.
- Take adequate rest between sets of exercises and between repe·tition exercises.
- Do not exercise in hot or humid conditions.
- Do not exercise (or at the very least limit or modify your exercise routine) if you are going through a relapse.
- Do not launch into the hardest exercise routine you can find without preparation. Start gently and work gradually up to the harder exercises. Short bouts of exercises done several times a day are better than one mammoth session.
- Avoid exercises that call for direct pressure on a spastic muscle. Spastic muscles are best exercised by stretching (but stop at once if a spastic muscle goes into spasm during exercise and wait for the spasm to subside before continuing).
- Drink plenty of liquid after exercising to avoid dehydration. The liquid should be mineral water or fruit juice ideally – but certainly never tea or coffee.

The dangers that over-exercising can do are now much better known than they once were. When international athletes such as

Sebastion Coe were young everyone thought that only raw steaks and constant training produced record-breakers. The fact that athletes, including Seb Coe, also kept on going down with mysterious viruses the whole time did not seem relevant. But we now know different.

Studies in North America in the last few years have shown that too much training – that is, intensive and sustained training over many years – can actually weaken the immune system. Scientists in Washington, for example, found that athletes were twice as likely to suffer from stomach bugs, respiratory diseases and skin complaints as non-athletes.

Canadian scientists now say that there is probably an optimum level of exercise for everyone. In other words exercise only works up to a certain point and then it becomes counter-productive. It makes you worse. No one knows what that 'balance point' is yet but experts are trying hard to find out. It is probably different for each person but the significant thing is that while moderate exercise is good and necessary over-doing it can definitely be dangerous.

Jenny is a dramatic, and tragic, example of what can happen that brings the point very much to home. For Jenny is a patient of mine. A former world-class athlete she is presently so crippled with MS she can hardly move. Cruelly struck down on the eve of a promising international career, Jenny, now 33, was ordered to eat huge amounts of protein like steak and train till she dropped in order to maintain peak fitness. It took her to the Great Britain junior team and to winning races against the best the Americans, Russians and Germans could put against her. But it has come close to destroying her.

Jenny has a mountain to climb just to be able to walk again (and she's determined to do it despite the severity of her symptoms) but she might never have had to face the climb in the first place if she hadn't been pushed so hard so young.

Of course, Jenny's case is exceptional but it is a warning to athletes everywhere nevertheless. All things in moderation, including exercise, is good advice to anyone. My own experience has led me to work out a routine that is very successful in allowing people with MS to exercise to maximum benefit and without exhausting themselves.

So if you are going to do any exercise try to remember *'Susie's tips for healthy exercise'*.

Tips for healthy exercise

- Exercise in cool (not cold) conditions. Hot or humid temperatures make MS symptoms worse. (So remember, always avoid having a hot bath.)
- Have a glass of mineral water or dilute fruit juice to hand to sip between exercises.
- Dress in loose, comfortable clothes and do without shoes if you can
- Always start with a gentle warm-up period first. Body squats or calf lifts are good for this.
- Do exercises in blocks of no more than ten with rest periods in between, even if for only a few seconds. For example, if you do ten calf lifts rest for say five seconds before doing another ten, rest for five seconds, another ten, rest and so on.
- Do only as much as you feel you can comfortably manage. If you feel worse after exercising you have done too much. It is much better to under-exercise in MS than over-exercise.
- Be consistent. Don't change your routine wildly just because you feel particularly good one day. Learn to monitor yourself and gauge your responses for maximum consistency. For example, if you normally swim four lengths of the pool but one day feel tired after only two then stop at two. Don't push yourself beyond the limits your body is telling you. Similarly with walking. If walking a quarter of a mile drains you when normally you would walk half a mile don't worry about it. Stop, and tell yourself that tomorrow you'll be fine. You have nothing to 'prove' by going on when your body is saying 'stop' and will probably feel a lot worse if you do.
- Listen to you body. Your body talks to you. Use your intuition, in other words, to find out if you are overdoing it. Your body wll tell you.

back
and spine

Your back, which means your spine together with all the large muscles and tissues attached to it, is arguably one of the most vital parts of your body – which also explains why this is the longest chapter in the book! Not only does your back hold you upright but it controls your overall posture – the way you stand and walk.

Good posture is important for more reasons than the obvious one of it not being very convenient to go around lop-sided. If our posture is good our muscles don't have to work as hard, our breathing is likely to be deeper and less strained, our blood stronger and more full of oxygen, our immune system more effective and we will feel more balanced, energetic and healthier generally.

Few people really understand how much posture affects our health in all sorts of ways, many of them unseen and unrealised most of the time.

Poor posture can cause problems not only with our backs, hands, arms and legs – all obvious enough perhaps – but less obvious parts of our body too such as ears, eyes, brain, throat, mouth, blood, bladder and bowels. It can also be responsible for a whole range of so-called 'psychosomatic' complaints common in people with MS from tiredness, depression and headaches to poor breathing, constipation and incontinence.

Sue is a good example. She came to see me a few days after she'd been involved in a car accident. Though she'd had MS for some years her symptoms were mild. Her legs were affected but not too badly. When she came to see me she could not walk at all and was in some distress. It seemed as if the accident, in which she hadn't been injured, had caused her to have a serious relapse.

She told me she was suffering from uncontrollable bouts of crying for no apparent reason, had lost all her appetite and felt overwhelming tiredness. The thought of going out, still less driving, was too daunting for words.

When I examined her I found clear signs of her back having gone into spasm – that is, the muscles of her back were tight and hard. She then admitted she had indeed been suffering back spasms since the accident but had assumed this was a symptom of MS.

Of course, it wasn't MS to blame but the accident. Five sessions of therapy later Sue was back to her old self again, appetite back and depression lifted.

The point about this story is not just how easy it is to blame MS for non-MS causes but how a physical problem with the back can cause such wide-ranging symptoms, affecting mind and emotions as well as the body. Sue was quite probably affected more than most because of her MS but anyone, including someone fully fit, could have suffered in much the same way.

The problem of poor posture is not one confined just to people with MS. Most people spend a lifetime with a body that is unbalanced. The fact is that these days most of us hold ourselves badly most of the time – the result of poor eating and living habits, lack of exercise, wearing the wrong shoes, sitting around too much and not sitting properly when we do sit.

All these things lead to muscle tightness and imbalances that in turn create abnormal weight distribution and stresses and strain on other, hidden, parts of the body – often far from the root of the problem.

The work we do, our temperament, the genes we were born with and diseases we catch or have can all affect our posture. But posture is something it is possible to do a very great deal to correct, regardless of what might have caused us to be the way we are (though some problems, such as inner ear infection that can cause a loss of balance, may need other treatment as well).

The important thing is to realise this and not rush off to the doctor for a drug at the first sign of tension or anxiety. Not knowing any better, he or she is likely to prescribe you drugs such as 'muscle relaxants', 'antidepressants' or 'tranquillisers' – none of which should be a first resort treatment and all of which have side-effects, some of them serious. (If you want to know more about drug treatments for MS and their dangers I recommend you read the excellent *The Natural Way with MS* by Richard Thomas, Element Books, UK/USA, 1995)

The main point of the exercises in this chapter is to help you correct and maintain good posture without drugs of any sort. This is done by following a programme of massage, muscle-stretching and strengthening, and exercise reinforced with reflexology.

The back and its connecting tissue needs to stay supple to work properly but lack of exercise and fatigue can soon harden tissue, reducing the flow of blood and lymph and so vital nutrients don't reach the parts they should. This chapter will also tell you what nutritional support you need. Together with massage and exercises it will help provide the answer your back needs to become fully fit and mobile again.

Ideal posture

The ideal back is not one that is ramrod straight. Curves are natural and normal. In fact, the spine has four natural curves – but they should be gentle and upright curves. A good back should have the right balance of curves for best performance and to avoid strain on muscles and joints.

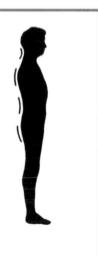

Common back problems

The illustration on the previous page is an example of good posture. But the ideal is seldom reality, as we all know, and most people I see have a variety of abnormalities that need correcting to allow the body to work at maximum efficiency and avoiding unnecessary stress and strain on connecting joints and muscles. Height plays a significant part in posture but the most common abnormalities I see associated with MS are: kyphosis, lordosis, 'flat back', 'sway back' and scoliosis.

Kyphosis

Kyphosis means a spine with exaggerated outward and inwards curves: the upper (thoracic) spine curves out too much – usually producing 'round shoulders', a 'flat chest' and an extended neck with the head coming too far forward – and the lower (lumbar) spine curves in too much, producing a very 'hollow' back (see right). This is the most common postural problem and it is often seen in people confined to a wheelchair or who spend most of their time sitting.

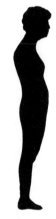

Kyphosis posture

For people in wheelchairs the problem is sometimes that they have developed kyphosis because of the soft back-padding of the chair they spend most of their time in. Their backs have become moulded to the shape of the padding, producing an unhealthy kyphotic shape where none was probably there in the first place.

■ Correcting kyphosis

Kyphosis puts pressure on the lungs and compresses the digestive system. This can not only affect a person's breathing capacity, sometimes leading to tingling and numbness in fingers from the shortage of oxygen to the tissues, asthma and other respiratory problems, but also result in constipation, incontinence and depression. Treatment concentrates on deep-breathing and posture correcting exercises.

■ Exercise 1

Placing a stick under your chin straighten your shoulders, pulling them back slowly but firmly. Your neck muscles will feel pulled and stretched but persevere without straining. Do only as much as feels comfortable as overtaxing the neck muscles will only make the problem worse.

■ Exercise 2

Stand or sit against a wall with your shoulders and upper back touching the wall. Stretch your arms above your head and touch the wall. Noting how easily your hands touch the wall above your head will give you a very good idea of how bad your posture is: if you can touch the wall easily it is good, if not it is a lot less good! Keep doing this as often as possible wherever possible. It will strengthen your back and shoulders muscles as well as help straighten your spine.

Note: People in wheelchairs should make sure they have a good solid back to their wheelchair and that they sit right back into the seat and sit up straight when they do this exercise.

Lordosis

Lordosis is a posture in which the lower spine is curved excessively inwards and, again, can be due to sitting too much or standing too long with the knees locked backwards (see right). It is commonly associated with weak stomach muscles and tight back muscles.

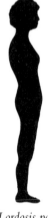

Lordosis posture

■ Correcting lordosis

Stand 'tall' when standing but relax the knees, don't force them back. Stand with the pelvis tilted slightly forward and the stomach muscles gently pulled in. Tuck the chin in. This will lengthen the back of the neck when standing and help reduce the 'poked forward' look common in lordosis. Exercises for strengthening stomach muscles will also help and these are shown later.

Flat back posture

Flat back means largely what it says: the pelvis is tilted too far forward, there is no curve of the lower spine and the muscles of the bottom are wasted, producing the characteristic 'flat' look. It is also common for people with flat backs to have round shoulders (see left).

■ Correcting a flat back

Whenever you sit down straighten your legs out in front of you. This will not only stretch your hamstrings, which are usually tight in this condition, but help accentuate the curve of the lower back. Also clench the muscles of your bottom as often as you can to help strengthen them. A lumbar support cushion or roll will also help. These are available from a variety of sources these days, including mail order.

Flat back posture

Sway back posture

In a sway back posture the entire lower back, including the pelvis and upper thighs are held forward so the upper body appears to lean backwards. The shoulders are usually rounded and the chin stuck out (see right). It is a posture common in people who are very flexible and the cause is mainly weak hips. It is sometimes mistaken for lordosis, though it is quite different.

Sway back posture

■ Correcting a sway back

When standing try to transfer your body weight onto the balls of the feet rather than the heels and pull your chin in. This will help lengthen the neck and lift some of the weight off the hips. You will also need to do hip and bottom muscle-strengthening exercises.

Scoliosis

Scoliosis is a sideways curvature or twist of the spine and is usually the result of habitually poor posture, though it can be inherited (see right). The effect is the same if you stand with your full weight on one foot and force your shoulders in that direction without actually turning. It is common in varying degrees in many people and characteristically produces different leg lengths.

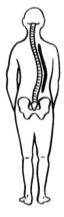

■ Correcting scoliosis

In severe cases a special lift fitted into a shoe will help the problem (though it must be done by someone qualified such as a podiatrist) but most people are not badly enough affected to need this sort of artificial aid and can help themselves quite easily by regularly stretching the muscles of the hips and trunk. Always try this first before resorting to artificial aids if you can.

I had a problem myself with muscle spasm pulling my spine and giving me backache. My right side was always very tight and I had great difficulty doing side-bending exercises as a result. I also had problems with my back when driving and used a lumbar cushion to stop my back aching during a long drive. One day, a colleague, another physical therapist, pointed out to me that I had a slight sideways curve to my spine.

I had been completely unaware of it until then and had always put the problem down to yet another inevitable result of MS. I walk with a stick, and have done so for years, so obviously what had happened is that over time the constant uneven walking had shortened and tightened my back muscles.

Needless to say, I immediately started on a short course of physical therapy involving me having the muscles of my lower back stretched. After about four sessions I found I could not only do side-bends comfortably but no longer needed the lumbar cushion in the car. I could also drive without getting backache. So I know at first hand just how important it is to stretch, even if you are fit and don't have any obvious aches and pains. The trouble is that often enough we 'learn to live with' the problem when we needn't have it in the first place.

It's also important to say at this point that although I have given an introduction to posture, working out whether or not you have a postural problem and what to do about it is not really best done on your own. I would always advise seeking professional help such as that from a qualified osteopath, chiropractor, physiotherapist, physical therapist or massage therapist. Other specialists in postural assessment are teachers of The Alexander Technique, Conductive Education (the 'Peto work') and the Feldenkrais Method.

Once you have discovered, though, that your posture is likely to be the cause of some of your problems you are on the road to doing something to relieve them. Any one of the above therapists is sure to be able to help you but you may simply decide, once you've got your 'diagnosis', you'd rather help yourself. In that case the following combination of massage and special exercises for the back will produce most benefit.

Massage for backs

For this you will obviously need a willing partner unless you would rather go to a therapist specializing in therapeutic massage. A properly-trained physical therapist or massage therapist will be able to carry out the sort of 'deep tissue massage', as it is known, that will help quickest but a good and sympathetic partner can be just as effective over a longer period if you'd rather not go to a therapist.

If you can find someone willing to do it for you the first thing is to make sure they use a good oil. Massage is only really effective if the person massaging uses oil so that their hands slide easily over your skin. Baby oil is excellent but grapeseed oil, available in most good stores, is best. For an even better effect add an essential oil to the 'base' oil (see box 'Essential oils for back massage').

Ask the person doing the massaging to begin the massage using light strokes. This allows you to relax and them to find any particular areas of tenderness and assess the general state of your back.

Essential oils for back massage

Essential oils are concentrated oils extracted from plants and not only are they said to have specific therapeutic qualities but they smell delicious too. Massage with essential oils is usually known as aromatherapy and is available from specially-trained therapists for a variety of complaints from spasm to stress.

For self-help home use it is enough to know that essential oils – readily available in almost any pharmacist, healthfood, beauty and gift shop these days – will add that extra luxury to the massage experience no matter what oil you use! But for best effect choose one or more from the following list:

Oil Action
■ **Lavender** A powerful but very safe decongestant, antidepressant and anti-infectant said to have a major calming, soothing and relaxing effect. Probably the single best all-purpose oil.

■ **Geranium** Stimulates the lymphatic system (and so supports the immune system), improves the circulation, and is a kidney tonic and overall 'balancer'.

■ **Rosemary** A stimulant said to be particularly effective for the central nervous system, brain and respiratory system, and as an antidote to fatigue.

■ **Evening primrose** Useful as a support for evening primrose oil taken internally (by capsule) as a dietary supplement.

Quality
With essential oils, as most things these days, you only get what you pay for. Very cheap oils tend to be low in purity and therefore low in efficacy. It's worth paying a bit more for oils of known quality. A good health shop or therapist should be able to help you.

How to use essential oils properly
It is best not to use essential oils undiluted because their effect can be very powerful. Most people find that the best way to use them is to dilute just two or three drops in about a teaspoonful (5ml) of neutral 'base' or 'carrier' oil such as grapeseed. It is also better to make sure oils are warmed to at least room temperature before using.

The basic back massage

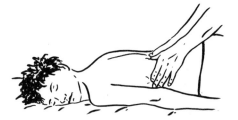

This a superficial massage and is the technique to use when you start a back massage. The palms of the hands should be used flat to stroke upwards along the back muscles either side of the spine towards the head.

Once you are both familiar with each other the massage can become more positive. The person massaging should increase the pressure of his or her strokes so that any slight discomfort should feel as if it is doing good rather than damage – such as in 'Oh, yes, that's good.' In fact guiding the person doing the massage with the odd comment like that is usually very useful. It aids the communication that is so important between the helper and the helped.

If the pressure ever becomes too painful ask the person massaging to go easier and use lighter, quicker movements instead.

Acupressure massage for the back

According to the Japanese art of shiatsu ('finger pressure'), there are special pressure 'points' in the muscles running down the back on either side of the spine (known as the 'erector spinal muscles'). The points run from just below the shoulder-blade down as far as the small of the back and pressure or light massage applied to them very effectively relaxes, tones and strengthens these important muscles.

Exercises for the back

Before doing any of the following exercises for the back it is important to stretch first to help prepare the muscles for work and to reduce the chance of stiffness and soreness afterwards. A massage beforehand obviously helps but a good stretch is useful even if you have already had a massage. Many of the exercises, such as 'The Cat', originated in yoga and so you may also find them called by other, usually animal, names in yoga.

■ The Cat stretch

Kneel as in the diagram below left, with your knees directly under your hips, arms straight down and head right up. Breathe in and let your spine curve downwards, shoulder blades pulled together. Hold for a second and breathe out, tucking your head down below your shoulders and arching your back upwards (below right). Repeat three or four times.

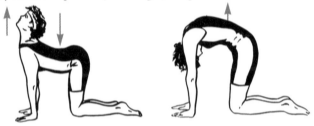

'The Cat' stretch exercises

■ Lower back release

Kneel as in diagram right and lie forward, arms out in front and the top of the feet flat on the floor. Make sure you are comfortable and relaxed. Now gently drop your lower back

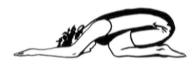

Lower back release

and backside between your feet towards the floor.

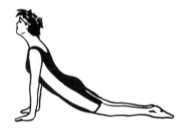

■ Extension stretch/spinal flexion

Placing your hands flat on the floor, move your legs out straight behind you and push yourself up, arms straight, to arch your back as in diagram left.

Extension stretch/spinal fexion

■ Lower back stretch

Sitting on the floor, stretch one leg out in front of you and bend the other inwards towards your groin. Place both hands on the out-stretched leg and bend forward, pushing your hands down the leg towards your foot. Bend forward in degrees, holding each stretch for

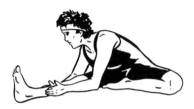

about eight seconds before stretching forward again. Increase the stretch by bending your toes towards you. Change legs and repeat the exercise.

Lower back stretch
Caution: Do not do this exercise if you have a curvature (kyphosis) of the upper spine.

■ Advanced back stretch

A progression from the above exercise. Putting both legs out in front of you, toes bent up, and with your hands flat on the floor beside you (taking the weight of your body off your lower spine), bend forward as far as you can to a count of

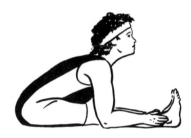

Advanced back stretch

eight (see diagram right). I have found that many people with MS have difficulty doing this exercise without first having extensive deep tissue massage and lumbar stretching from an experienced therapist to release the restriction and tension in the lower back area.

■ Lower back release

Lie on your back with your knees bent and your hands flat on the floor. Press the small of your back into the floor and hold this pressure

Lower back release

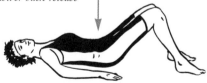

for up to ten seconds before relaxing (see left). This is a wonderful exercise for lower back pain.

■ Spinal release stretch

Still lying on your back, lift your knees off the floor by holding them with your hands and pulling back (see diagram at top next page).

Spinal release stretch

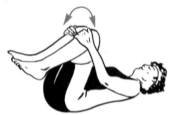

Keeping your knees at right angles to your hips slowly push them first one way and then the other to rotate the hips.

■ Pelvis and lower back release

Lie on your back and with your hands holding your knees lift your feet off the floor. Let one leg drop gently outwards towards the floor and then bring the other leg over to join it (see right). Now move this second leg back to the upright position and drop it on the opposite side of you and bring the first leg over to join it. This exercise should be done as one slow, continuous movement, without stopping.

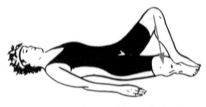

Pelvis and lower back release

■ Knee hug stretch

Lying down, bring one knee up and clasp it with both hands. Pull it towards your chest at the same as bringing your head down (see left). Change knees and repeat the exercise. This exercise is particularly good for the muscles of the hips, bottom and lower back.

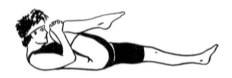

Knee hug stretch

■ Spinal rotation stretch

Again lying straight out on your back, lift one leg over the other so that it touches the floor on the other side (you will need to bend it slightly to do this). Place the hand nearest on top of the knee and press gently downwards. Make sure the other shoulder stays on the floor

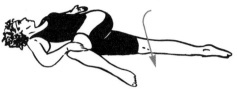

Spinal rotation stretch

with the arm outstretched. So if you lift your right leg over your left (as left), press down on your right knee with your left hand while your right shoulder stays flat on the floor and your right arm is outstretched. Now turn your head to look at your outstretched hand. You can increase the pressure, and the benefit, by making your knee resist the pressure of the hand pushing it down. Do this to a count of ten and relax. Repeat the exercise on the opposite side (left leg to right side and so on).

■ Buttock strengthening

Lie on your stomach and bend one leg at right angles to the floor. Pushing your pelvis into the floor, tighten your buttocks and lift your bent leg

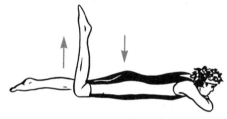

Buttock strengthening

bent leg up off the ground (see above). Keep your toes bent down but be careful not to arch your back. Hold for a few seconds and relax. Change legs and repeat the exercise.

■ Pelvic lift

Again on your back, lie with your arms straight and your hands flat on the floor, knees bent. Pushing down on your hands and arms, and clenching your buttock muscles, lift your pelvis as far up as you can

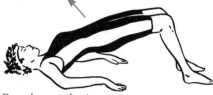

Buttock strengthening

without arching your back (see left). Hold for a few seconds and relax. This exercise also helps strengthen the bladder (see next chapter).

Chest stretching and breathing exercise

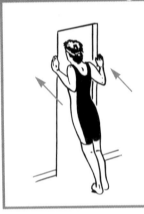

The following simple exercise is excellent for stretching the muscles of the chest (and the shoulders) and helping with breathing. Stand or sit in a doorway, place your hands on the doorposts on either side at shoulder height and then lean forward gently. You should feel a stretch mainly in the chest area. Hold the stretch for five seconds and then return to the upright position. Do this ten times.

■ Back exercises for the immune system

As I've mentioned earlier, the immune system is heavily involved in MS and an important part of the immune system is a secondary system known as 'the lymphatic system'. The lymphatic system consists of a network of tiny channels that run through the body rather like blood vessels and carry a fluid known as 'lymph'. Its job is to clear out of the body toxins and other unwanted waste material mopped up by the blood supply.

Unlike blood, though, which is moved rapidly round the body by the heart, lymph has no such independent pump to move it around. It relies on the natural movement of the body to move it. So someone who does not or cannot exercise, such as someone in a wheelchair, is likely to have unwanted toxins lingering around in the system, lowering resistance and increasing the likelihood of disease.

So it is easy to see how very important it is that everyone, but particularly those with MS confined to a wheelchair, exercise as regularly as possible. An alternative to exercising to keep the lymphatic system healthy is massage. A good massage can have much the same effect as exercise – but, again, it must be done often.

The following exercises not only have an envigorating effect on the muscles of the back but stimulate the lymphatic system too.

■ Back and body tapping

Tapping, or 'body percussion', is a technique well-known in the Orient where it has links with acupuncture and acupressure (or shiatsu). In the East it is commonly used to tone up and envigorate the body and its internal organs by following what are known as 'energy flow lines' or 'meridians'. But its benefits are now also becoming better known and followed in the West.

Start by lightly tapping either side of the neck and shoulders with loosely-clenched fists. Do this for about half a minute only. Then lean forward and, reaching up behind your back as far as possible, do the same thing up and down either side of your spine and onto your buttocks (see below). Make the tapping stronger as you get used to it.

Continue the tapping down the side of your arms and up to your shoulders, coming back into the upright position as you do so. Then do the same down the inside of your legs and up the outside to your buttocks.

End by vigorously tapping up your body, over your chest and onto your breast-bone just below the collar-bone. The tapping on your breast should be more of a beating than a tapping, in fact. Imagine you are Tarzan (me Jane!) and you've got it about right. You can do a Tarzan yell when doing this, if you like. It helps relieve tension and stress of many sorts.

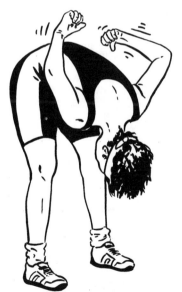

This chest-beating is most important. It stimulates the thymus gland which is vital part of the body's immune system.

The final step is to rap and tap all over your head. It'll help 'wake your brain'.

Tapping is best done first

Body tapping

thing in the morning. It is simple enough to carry it out on yourself but it can also effectively be done for you by someone else.

■ Ball rolling

The simplest way to massage your own back is to buy any of the number of devices now on the market, from wooden balls on the end of a stick to an electrically-operated massager, that do most of the work for you. But an even simpler way of reaching your back without contorting yourself too much if you don't want to go to any expense is to trap a tennis ball or any ball of similar size against a wall with your back (see right). Press the ball against the wall and simply move up and down and around it. This, too, will not only give you a good all-over massage but help relieve tension. It can also be done in a wheelchair.

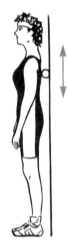

Ball rolling

■ Back rocking

This is a variation on the above. Rather than roll yourself against a ball, lie down on your back on a hard but comfortable surface, curl yourself up by holding your knees tightly in your arms and then simply rock backwards and forwards and from side to side as if you were a ball yourself (see left). The rolling will become easier and the movement smoother as the spine loosens up. This exercise is also really good for toning the stomach muscles.

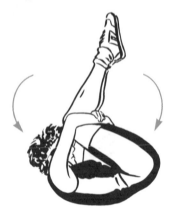

Back rocking

■ Back stretching

As usual, end with a good stretching exercise. The following is both easy and effective: find a sturdy chair and hold onto it as shown in the diagram on the following page. Stand with your feet apart and your back as flat as you can make it. You

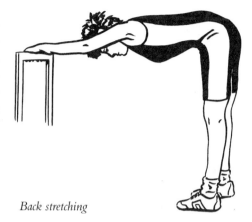

Back stretching

may feel some pulling in the muscles in the back of your legs, especially if your hamstrings are tight, but this is normal so persevere. If it is too painful at first bend your kneess slightly to relax your legs. You should be able to feel the stretch in your back and, perhaps, also in your shoulders.

Back and upper body strengthening exercises for those with poor upper body strength

Quite the easiest and most pleasant way to increase the strength of your back and upper body – and not only if you use a wheelchair either – is to rock gently back and forth in a rocking chair. Rocking makes you use your upper body and legs and gives you the strength you need to rise up from the sitting position. (If you find the exercise too easy sit slightly away from the back of the chair to make it harder). So if you haven't already got a rocking chair make sure you put it on your Christmas or birthday list!

An enjoyable alternative to rocking in a rocking chair is to swing on a swing (but make sure it is strong enough to take your weight!). Swinging not only increases upper body strength but leg strength and coordination. Yet more alternatives are the following exercises:

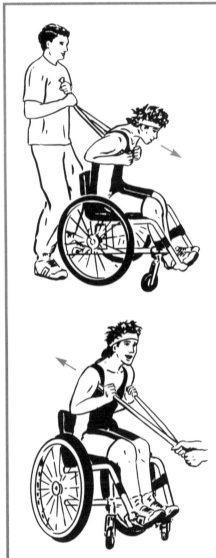

■ Seated abdominal curl

You will need a helper for this. Ask your helper to hold both ends of a stretch band behind you. Loop the band around your chest, cross your arms over your chest and with your elbows pressed lightly against your sides slowly bend forward as far as possible (see left). If you find your balance is bad or too difficult to keep support yourself by holding the arm-rests of the chair.

■ Back straighten

Loop the stretch band around your upper back so that it fits up under your armpits. Bend forward and have your helper hold the ends of the band at your waist level. Holding the band in place under your armpits by pressing your elbows into your sides and gripping the band with both hands as in the illustration left sit backwards against the pull of the band until your back touches the back of the seat. Make sure you keep your head and back straight. Don't let your head bend back. If your back musces are very weak you may not need the band. You may find that the force of gravity alone is enough to give you benefit.

Reflexology for the back

As the diagram below shows, the area of the feet that corresponds to the spine in reflexology is the length of the inside of both feet from the base of the big toe to the heel. There are a total of 29 different major bones (or *vertebrae*) in the spine and each of these has its corresponding place on the feet.

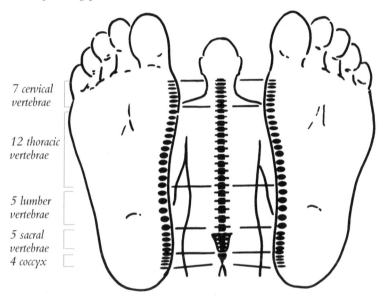

7 cervical vertebrae

12 thoracic vertebrae

5 lumber vertebrae

5 sacral vertebrae

4 coccyx

The spine as represented in reflexology

To help the spine a reflexologist will apply pressure along the inside of the soles of both feet. This is to promote not only the movement of the spine itself but the web of nerves, muscles and soft tissue attached to it and running to and from it, including the blood supply and lymphatic system. It will also help with the lungs and respiratory system. The diagrams on the next page show you the specific areas on the foot likely to help both your upper and lower back most.

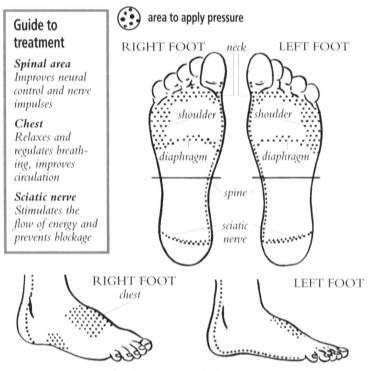

Reflexology points for back problems

Guide to treatment

Spinal area
Improves neural control and nerve impulses

Chest
Relaxes and regulates breathing, improves circulation

Sciatic nerve
Stimulates the flow of energy and prevents blockage

Reflexology and deep breathing

One of the biggest faults of people with MS in my experience is shallow breathing. Shallow breathing is the result of not breathing properly and it means stale air, full of poisonous carbon dioxide, stays in the lungs instead of leaving them, producing a loss of energy and worse illness (see box 'Why breathing properly is vital for good health').

A major cause of shallow breathing is stress. Massaging the balls of the feet, the front of the toes and halfway down the feet helps stimulate the lungs and diaphragm by inducing a feeling of relaxation which reduces stress and automatically improves circulation to all parts of the body.

Combined with relaxed deep breathing exercises (see chapter 5, pages 68-70), reflexology can quickly help the whole body to become fully oxygenated.

Why breathing properly is vital for good health

The respiratory system is the body's breathing mechanism. It consists basically of the nose, mouth, throat and lungs and is closely involved with the body's circulatory system, the system that circulates blood throughout the body. So another key organ is the heart.

The respiratory and circulatory systems work together to bring oxygen to every cell in the body. Oxygen is the single most important element we need. Without oxygen we would quickly die. Oxygen comes into our bodies in the air we breathe and is passed into our bloodstream through our lungs via tiny air 'sacs' known as *alveoli*.

The bloodstream takes the oxygen to the smallest cell where it combines with nutrients entering the body through the digestive system in the form of food and drink to produce energy – the fuel of life. So it is easy to see how vitally interconected our respiratory system is with both our circulatory and digestive systems.

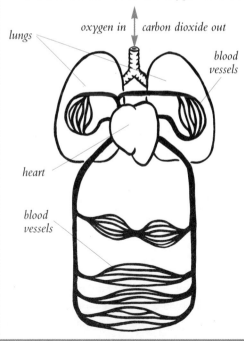

lungs

oxygen in | *carbon dioxide out*

blood vessels

heart

blood vessels

How the circulatory and respiratory systems connect up

Using reflexology successfully

It is important to experience reflexology properly to benefit fully. Some people find it can be painful at first and others find it tickles – so start by doing these few simple exercises to relax your feet. You'll need someone to help you so choose a sympathetic partner.

Sit or lie so you can comfortably put your feet on your partner's lap. A bed is the best place, with your partner sitting in front of the soles of your feet.

First, get your partner to massage talcum powder into your feet and get you both used to the idea of them being worked on. Ask him or her to start by gently pressing your feet and to get gradually firmer as they get used to the feel of you.

The next step is to relax the feet by stretching them (stretching comes into many of the exercises in MS). Ask your helper to grasp both feet above the back of the heels, supporting the ankle joint, and lean slowly backwards, stretching the legs from the hip. Ask your helper not to pull. Tell them to let the weight of their body do the work. This exercise also stretches the lower back and hips and helps relieve any tension in that area.

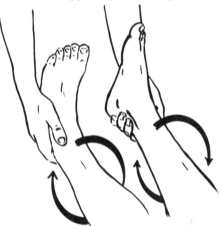

Ankle rocking

Don't worry if the legs appear to lengthen a fraction. This is normal.

Next, still holding both feet by the heels, gently rock the ankles from side to side (see diagram above).

A very important pressure point on the feet for relaxation is the hollow in the centre of the sole of the foot that corresponds to the solar plexus (see diagram on next page). The solar plexus is the network of nerves more or less in the centre of the body (behind the stomach but in front of the diaphragm) and is a part of the involuntary or 'autonomic' nervous system, the system that regulates the way organs such as the heart, lungs and stomach function.

Putting pressure on the solar plexus point on the feet (see diagram below) should be done at the same time as carrying out the following breathing exercise:

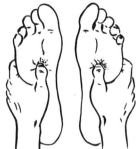

■ Ask your partner to press down on the point with his or her thumbs for a few seconds and to push your feet towards you while you breathe in.

■ Breathe out while your partner gently pulls your toes towards him or her and then lets them go.

Pressing the solar plexus point

■ Do this four or five times, after which your feet should feel relaxed and happy for anyone to touch them without feeling ticklish or painful.

Hardly anybody experiences reflexology who doesn't say how wonderfully relaxed it makes them feel. Whatever else reflexology does it is certainly relaxing – and this, of course, is why it's so good for MS.

Nutritional support

Chronic back pain – that is, back pain over a period – is not mainly, of course, a nutritional matter but the right sort of nutritional support can help with back pain just as it can help with most ailments if tailored correctly to the individual needing treatment. For example, pains in most joints, including the back, can sometimes be a symptom of a deficiency in the mineral manganese so taking manganese supplements could help. The recommended daily amount is 5–25mg.

Manganese normally enters our diet from the soil our food grows in. Good food sources of manganese are green leafy vegetables, bran, wheat, kelp, nuts, seeds and fruit, especially pineapple. The trouble is that often these days over-farming drains the minerals from the soil so that not enough get into the food chain for our needs. Manganese deficiency can also be the result of eating too many sugar products and other refined and processed foods low in manganese. Another cause is not having enough of the right digestive enzymes in our body. These naturally decrease as we get older. My research, using hair mineral analysis tests, suggests that almost everyone is enzyme deficient these days.

Supplementation with manganese is best done with a multivitamin because minerals and vitamins work best together. For advice on taking digestive enzymes it is best to see a qualified nutritional therapist.

A final note on back pain

Back pain is not to be treated lightly. Severe back pain can be extremely serious and if your pain is this bad consult either your doctor or a specialist in treating back pain such as a qualifed ostoeopath, chiropractor or physical therapist as soon as possible. Most important of all, never attempt difficult manipulation yourself or let anyone else do it to you unless they are properly trained and qualified to do so. An excellent book on back problems if you would like to look further into this important subject is *The Back and Beyond* by Dr Paul Sherwood (Arrow Books, UK, 1992).

bladder and bowels

Bladder and bowel problems are very common in MS. Bladder problems range from not being able to pass water, passing water frequently or hesitantly, to an urgent need to pass water. The main problem with bowels is constipation and stool inconsistency on the one hand and complete lack of bowel control on the other.

Of the two, bladder problems are the more usual as well as the more serious because not being able to pass water can lead to infection and pain. Bladder problems can also lead to cystitis and, in men, problems of the prostate. But constipation is not to be taken lightly either. It produces a buildup of toxins in the gut that can lead to a number of conditions linked to MS such as fatigue, bloatedness, a feeling of heaviness, lethargy, tiredness, depression and pain.

Both problems can, though, be caused by conditions nothing to do with MS. In Britain alone more than three million adults – one adult in every 15, but nearly one in three of elderly people – and half a million children are affected by 'urinary incontinence', as it is known, at some point in their lives. So it is important – as I am always pointing out – to look for other causes first.

For example, bladder problems can be caused by diabetes, allergies, kidney disease, candidiasis and, in men, enlargement of the prostate gland as well as by drugs commonly given to people with MS such as diuretics, benzodiazepines (valium, diazepam and so on), strong painkillers and some heart drugs (such as ACE inhibitors).

Bowel problems, on the other hand, are widespread throughout the western world these days largely as a result, it seems, of a combination of stressful lifestyles and a junk-food diet. One of the most common, and rapidly increasing, is irritable bowel syndrome (IBS) and that is now widely believed to be the combined result of stress and poor nutrition.

Bladder (or 'waterworks') and bowels are only loose descriptions of what is really the body's elimination system. Technically, the bladder is part of what is known as the urinary system and the bowels the digestive system (see pages 105 and 111). But their combined job is to eliminate the toxic waste products resulting from the conversion of what you eat and drink into the energy your body needs to function.

So the job of the urinary system (which consists of the bladder, ureter and urethra as well as the kidneys) is to eliminate the liquid waste product of the digestive system known as *urea*, the main substance in urine. The bowels (a general term for the lower half of the digestive system, including the small intestine, the large intestine or colon and the rectum) also contain some liquid but they are involved more in getting rid of solid waste or *faeces*.

Treatment for problems of the elimination system is a combination of things that are good for both bladder and bowels, such as what you eat and drink, and others are specifically for either bladder or bowels. These include special exercises and 'retraining' programmes.

Let's look first at the main problem area: the bladder.

Treating the bladder

No two people are alike and that includes people with MS. And because no two people are the same no two cases of MS are the same either. So successful treatment for the bladder is a matter of sensitively working out a combination of physical and dietary therapies most effective for you as an individual. Some you can do yourself but others you may need help with.

How the bladder works

The bladder sends urine to the urethra, the 'waste pipe' leading out of you, via two rings of muscles called sphincters. The first of these two rings prevents urine leaking out involuntarily. It is controlled by the autonomic nervous system *(see chapter 2)* and works automatically, without any conscious control on our part. But the second is normally under our conscious control. This is the muscle you relax when you urinate. As the urine starts to flow the muscles of your bladder (known as detrusor muscles) contract and this is what forces the urine out in a rush.

The most common type of incontinence is where the bladder muscles contract involuntarily, usually during the night when we are relaxed, causing a sudden – and mostly highly inconvenient! – need to urinate.

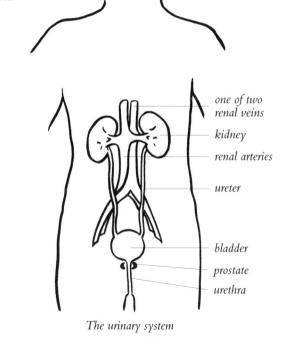

- one of two renal veins
- kidney
- renal arteries
- ureter
- bladder
- prostate
- urethra

The urinary system

Self help

Self-help treatment includes
- ■ pelvic floor exercises
- ■ bladder retraining
- ■ diet
- ■ nutritional support.

■ Pelvic floor exercises

These exercises are the same as those described in chapter 6 for back problems (see pages 87–92).

■ Bladder retraining programme

You can help 'retrain' your bladder by keeping a record of how much you drink, how much urine you pass and how often you pass it. The idea is that by keeping a record in this way you train yourself to extend the time between urinating. So, for example, if you find you are passing water every two hours try and extend the time so you pass water only every three hours. It requires an effort of will to suppress the need to pass water but it can be done.

Once you find you can remain 'dry' for the extra hour, extend the interval by a further half an hour, and so on, until you have regained control over yourself and are passing water at normal intervals of only every four or five hours or so.

■ Diet

The most important thing anyone can do with a bladder problem is to increase their intake of fluid, particularly of good, clean, fresh water. Cutting down on fluids does not mean, as many think, fewer trips to the toilet. On the contrary, what happens if you do not drink enough liquid during the day is that your urine becomes concentrated and not only smells strongly but can lead to infection developing in the bladder and the urge to pass water all the more.

People with MS should try and drink at least 1.5 to two litres of water a day, preferably filtered or bottled (still). Water is not only important for food digestion and elimination but is crucially involved in the temperature control of our bodies. Few people know that 62 per cent of an average adult's body weight and 75 per cent of a child's is water and that we lose about two litres of water every 24 hours – more if we exercise.

So drink plenty of water throughout the day. Sipping at regular intervals from a glass of water beside you or a small bottle is a good way of making sure you get enough. Don't wait until you feel thirsty. Dehydration has already set in by the time anyone feels thirsty.

Another important tip is not to drink copious amounts of liquid with food. By all means drink before a meal and after one but try not to drink during one, except to swallow any vitamin and mineral supplements you may be taking. Swamping food with fluid makes it too liquid. This means it not only flushes too quickly through the system – not letting the nutrients in the food be absorbed into the bloodstream – but it doesn't give the bowels the right amount of fibre. Bowels need fibre to function properly, that means regularly and smoothly.

Another good way to take in fluids healthily is to drink fruit juice. Freshly-prepared fruit juice is a wonderful start to any day and I certainly recommend it for anyone with MS, with or without a bladder problem. Cranberry juice is particularly good for helping any bladder problem, including cystitis.

Juicing your own fresh fruit – preferably organic if you can get it – is best but not always possible so make sure you buy only still (non fizzy) additive-free juices in glass bottles or card cartons. Juice degenerates or 'oxidizes' very quickly once it is extracted so look out for freshly-squeezed juice without any additives or preservatives if you can because this will be as close to doing your own juicing as you can.

You should be able to see bits of fruit in the juice if it is really fresh. But beware phrases on the bottles or cartons such as 'pasteurized', 'fresh', 'pure' or 'real juice'. None of them mean the juice is freshly squeezed and it is quite likely to contain additives such as acid, sugar, preservatives and pulp wash (produced by soaking the skins of the fruit in water and pulping it). Pasteurized is even worse and unfortunately a lot of fruit juice is pasteurized these days. As in milk, pasteurized means its nutritional content has been altered and reduced.

What about tea and coffee? A lot of people ask me this and the answer surprises some of them. I don't ban either. In moderation – which means no more than two or three cups (or one mugfull) a day – both tea and coffee can have benefits. The Institute of Optimum Nutrition in Britain recommends no more than a cup of coffee a day or three cups of tea.

For example, caffeine, the addictive stimulant in both tea and coffee, seems to be able to increase the effect of pain-killer drugs while tea is a good source of manganese, an essential mineral often deficient in people with MS. Herbal teas are also excellent body cleansers and strengtheners (see box 'Herbal tea remedies'). Both tea and coffee are natural diuretics. That is, they encourage the body to release fluid.

Herbal tea remedies

- **Indigestion and stomach-ache**
  peppermint, caraway, dill, fennel, lemon grass, lemon balm
- **Infections and colds**
  rose hip, coltsfoot, comfrey, aniseed, licorice, sage
- **Sleep-inducing and nerve-calming**
  chamomile, hops, lime, orange blossom, passion flower
- **General tonic**
  mint, rosemary, ginseng, raspberry, blackberry, strawberry leaf

Herb teas can be drunk either hot or cold. Ice teas need to be stronger to taste. For those who must have their tea sweet use honey rather than sugar.

The really bad news about tea and coffee, though, is that too much – and other caffeine-rich drinks such as hot chocolate and cola also – can trigger a whole range of unpleasant symptoms from anxiety, nervousness, depression, insomnia and shakiness to fatigue, tremors, palpitations, hypertension and restless legs at night. (Even decaffeinated tea and coffee is not much better because many manufacturers introduce other, equally harmful, chemicals during the decaffeinating process.)

Drinking too much tea and coffee with vegetables can also reduce by a third the amount of iron absorbed and cut the natural absorption of zinc.

Nutritional support

Bladder problems can be helped very effectively by careful control of what you eat and drink. For example, cutting out all white flour and white flour products as well as sugar and sugar products, including drinks with sugar in, and drinking between two and three litres (4-6 pints) of pure, clean water (filtered or bottled) a day will help your bladder work better and reduce the risk of getting common bladder infections.

You will also help your bladder by keeping to a diet that reduces animal fat to a minimum, that does not involve drinking too much alcohol and avoids all processed foods.

To help prevent infections like cystitis avoid washing the genital area with perfumed soaps and toiletries and wearing nylon underwear, tights or trousers.

Food supplements for a healthy bladder include zinc, vitamins A and C, and essential fatty acids such as oil of evening primrose. Calcium and magnesium supplements are also effective, especially if taken with extract of cranberry and acidophilus. The table below shows the right daily doses.

Daily supplements for bladder problems

Calcium/magnesium*	500mg calcium/200-400mg magnesium
Acidophilus**	2 capsules
Cranberry extract (powder)	5g
Beta carotene	15mg
Vitamin A	7,500iu
Evening Primrose Oil	up to 1500mg (best as 500mg capsules)

*Calcium/magnesium should be taken as a single supplement with two parts calcium to one part magnesium. The specialist suppliers listed at the end of this book should be able to help.
**Acidophilus capsules should be in the strength of four billion organisms per capsule at least. Capsules must be fresh and should be keep refrigerated at all times. Your specialist supplier will be able to advice you more on this.

Treatment from others

■ Physical therapy (massage and manipulation)

Massage and manipulation, especially of the lower back, can be very helpful for both bladder and bowel problems in MS. Again, the parts of chapter 6 detailing massage and manipulation for the lower back apply here also. Particularly helpful for bladder and bowel problems are the back stretching exercises.

However a word of caution here: if you think manipulation might help you it really is best to seek out the help of a properly trained and qualified therapist – not just for effectiveness but also for safety. Manipulating, even just stretching, the spine is highly dangerous and should only be done by someone who really knows what they are doing.

The same is not so true of massage but you will still normally get more benefit from someone properly trained than someone not.

Massage tip: Use the essential oil chamomile with your base oil. Chamomile has known anti-inflammatory properties that are particularly good for bowel and bladder problems.

■ Reflexology

Reflexology helps to promote the efficient working of the urinary system by assisting the detoxifying process and preventing and alleviating any blockages and infections that occur. The diagram on the next page shows you the areas on the feet that relate to the urinary system and bladder.

Guide to treatment

Diaphragm
*Regulates breathing
and aids relaxation*

**Head/brain, hypothalamus
and pineal gland**
Stimulates glandular function

Lower spine
*Relaxes muscles and stimulates
nerves to the bladder*

Bladder and kidneys
*Regulates elimination
of urine*

Adrenals
*Stimulates hormones
for water balance*

 area to apply pressure

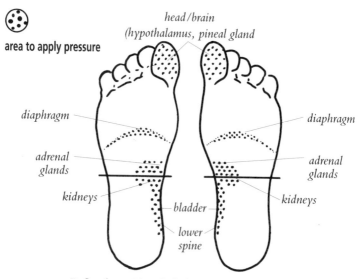

area to apply pressure

head/brain
(hypothalamus, pineal gland

diaphragm

diaphragm

adrenal
glands

adrenal
glands

kidneys

kidneys

bladder

lower
spine

Reflexology points for kidney and bladder problems

Treating the bowels

Bowel problems are not quite so common or so serious as bladder problems in MS but they are still quite bad enough. Constipation – being unable to pass stools or passing them only with great difficulty – is probably the most common complaint closely followed by incontinence. Incontinence of the bowel is not being able to control the bowels and is often associated with diarrhoea in MS.

Bowel problems can also be the result of poor muscle tone in the intestines from lack of exercise, fatigue and anxiety. Poor diet, especially lack of fibre, is also a cause as is sensitivity of the bowels to some foods, drugs (especially antidepressants, antacids, laxatives and iron tablets), and mental stress and depression. Inactivity and prolonged sitting, particularly in a wheelchair, can have a serious effect on the colon and elimination process, and is a major cause of constipation.

As with the bladder, successful treatment is a matter of finding out what works best in your case and tailoring treatment to your specific needs and responses. Again, you will probably find it is a combination of physical therapy and diet, and again some you can do yourself and others you may need the help of others.

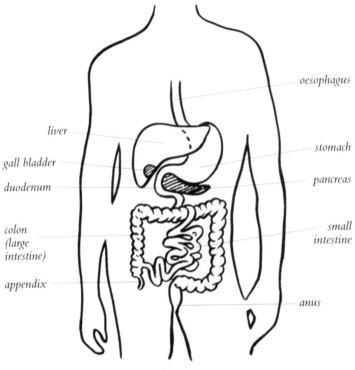

oesophagus

liver

stomach

gall bladder

pancreas

duodenum

colon
(large
intestine)

small
intestine

appendix

anus

The digestive system

Self-help

■ Exercise

Any exercise – especially in fresh air – is good for both bladder and bowels, especially those for the back in chapter 6.

■ Reflexology

Use the diagram on pages 115 to treat your own reflex points.

■ Diet

A common problem of people with MS is low energy from hypoglycaemia (low blood sugar) and this is often the result of poor diet coupled with bowel problems. Both constipation and diarrhoea are problems commonly experienced by people with MS and in both cases not enough nutrients get into the body's 'energy chain'.

For constipation

Eating plenty of wholegrains, vegetables, fruit, nuts, seeds and whole-meal flour products will give the bowels the level of dietary fibre it needs to stay heathy. The effect will be helped by cutting down or avoiding milk and dairy products, sugar, sweets, chocolates, cakes, white bread and white rice.

Another useful thing to do is increase your fluid intake by drinking at least two or three glasses of clean water. Tea is not good for constipation. It is a diuretic – which means it promotes dehydration and so encourage constipation. Long-term use of laxatives also, ironically, does the same (and not enough people know that!).

For diarrhoea

Diarrhoea is less common than constipation in MS but can have just as damaging effects unless treated. Prolonged diarrhoea can cause severe dehydration which is a serious condition.

Diarrhoea can be the result of food intolerance, digestive enzyme insufficiency and taking antibiotics over a long period as well as a symptom of irritable bowel syndrome (IBS).

A healthy stool should be solid, well-formed and float in the pan after being passed. The loose and usually runny stools that sink, common in diarrhoea, mean that there is an inadequate amount of bulk in the diet. If diarrhoea is ever the problem you need to drink plenty of good, clean water. Ironically, lack of fluid in the diet can actually bring on diarrhoea.

Nutritional support

Constipation can be a symptom of magnesium deficiency, especially in women who suffer from premenstrual syndrome (PMS) and those taking diuretic drugs (for high blood pressure, for example). Diuretic drugs commonly produce both magnesium and potassium deficiencies. A hair mineral analysis can show if any such deficiencies exist and if they do, the answer is to take a magnesium/potassium supplement. Taking vitamin C can also help as can acidophilus and soluble fibre. Peppermint oil can help with an irritable bowel. The table below gives the right doses to take.

If digestive enzyme deficiency is diagnosed as the cause of *diarrhoea*

Recommended daily supplements for bowel problems

Acidophilus	2 capsules
Soluble fibre	10-20g
Vitamin C	1-3g
If taking diuretic drugs	
Magnesium/potassium	200mg
If suffering from Irritable Bowel Syndrome (IBS)	
Peppermint oil	50mg (three times daily)

you will need to take special supplements but seek the help and advice of a qualified therapist. The best makers of supplements have a qualified nutritionist on the staff who is there to give such advice freely so I always recommend people to go only to suppliers who offer such a service. Their supplements are usually the best quality too. A list of recommended suppliers is at the end of this book.

Treatment from others

■ Physical therapy *(massage and manipulation)*

The same applies as for the bladder. An effective massage for the bowels, preferably using the oils listed in the box below, is to apply a gentle circular movement of the stomach and intestines – in other words, the whole of the area from the bottom of the rib-cage down to the pelvic bone or groin. Massage should be done in a circular and clockwise direction. This follows the direction the bowels lie and move.

Essential oils for the bowels

Oils	Good for
Chamomile	Diarrhoea and constipation
Cypress	Diarrhoea
Fennel	Constipation
Lavender	Diarrhoea
Marjoram	Constipation
Rosemary	Constipation

Note Essential oils for bowel problems should only be used individually. Do not mix the above oils except under expert guidance. That means an aromatherapist trained in the therapeutic use of oils (sometimes known as a 'clinical aromatherapist').

Reflexology

Manipulation of the areas shown in the diagram below will help a variety of bowel problems such asconstipation and diarrhoea as well as flatulence.

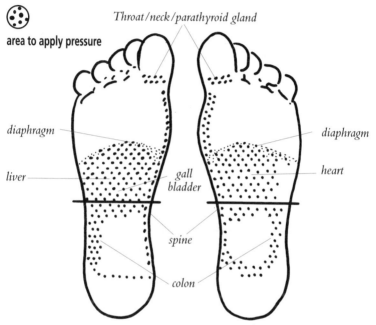

area to apply pressure

Throat/neck/parathyroid gland

diaphragm

diaphragm

liver

heart

gall bladder

spine

colon

Reflexology points for bowel problems

Guide to treatment

Diaphragm
Regulates breathing and promotes relaxation

Heart
Improves circulation

Throat/neck/parathyroid
Aids movement of food and regulates minerals necessary for peristalsis, relaxes neck

Spine
Stimulates nerves to the colon

Liver
Detoxifies blood

Gall bladder
Encourages bile release which assists fat digestion

Colon
Encourages waste elimination. Note: when massaging the colon area always make sure to apply pressure in a clockwise direction across both feet as shown.

legs and feet

Legs and feet show a variety of symptoms in people with MS, from feelings of tingling, numbness, heaviness, weakness, stiffness and pain to poor mobility and circulation, swelling, poor colour, spasm and restlessness. Walking can feel like you are trying to plough your way through heavy snow or water on the one hand or as if you are treading on eggs on the other.

All such symptoms are mostly due to a fault in the motor nervous system, the part of the nervous system that deals with the muscles. The cause is usually demyelination of the spinal cord rather than the brain so treatment includes work to the back as well as the legs and feet.

The most important treatment for problems of legs and feet is carrying out regular stretching exercises. These, together with special mobility and coordinating exercises, massage and manipulation to the back, legs and feet, reflexology, and dietary and nutritional support, can prove highly effective in helping to relieve the worst symptoms of MS in the legs and feet.

Stretching exercises for legs and feet

The importance of muscle-stretching exercises for people with MS cannot be over-emphasised – as I have tried to make very clear throughout this book. But stretching is particularly important when it comes to the muscles and ligaments of the legs.

Muscles that are not regularly exercised and stretched not only lose strength and mobility but become wasted and tight. What happens is that they become hard and tighter and this tightening happens very quickly, as anyone who has spent too long in bed knows only too well.

Legs hold the largest muscles of the body after the back and muscle contraction there can soon result in serious disability if correcting action is not taken at the earliest opportunity. Furthermore, deformity and distortion of leg muscles can cause more than just walking impairment. It can also affect the muscles of the rest of the body, particularly the muscles of the back, and, as described in chapter 6, this in turn can lead to all those other problems linked to posture and balance.

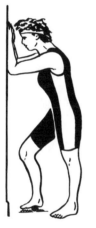

■ Stretching the whole leg

Stand close enough to a wall or some other strong support that you can lean against as in the illustration left. Placing a small, soft object under the arch of your foot (a rolled-up bandage is good), lean forward against the wall making sure your leg is straight and your heel on the floor. You should feel your leg muscles, particularly the outer leg muscle and calf, stretching evenly. Hold the stretch for up to ten seconds if you can and then relax.

The quickest way to stop the stretch if it is uncomfortable is simply to let your knee bend. This exercise is particularly good as a treatment for muscle spasms.

■ Stretching the thigh muscles

The thigh muscles are the largest and strongest muscles in the leg. To stretch them effectively:

- stand up straight with one hand on a chair or table for support
- bend one leg up behind you until you can grab hold of your foot

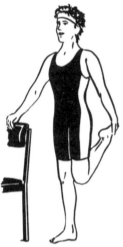

with your hand. Gently push your foot into your buttocks (see left). (If you can't manage to lift it high enough to grab on your own get someone to help you.) You should feel the thigh muscle (the large muscle on the top front of your leg) stretch.

● hold this position for ten seconds and let your leg drop. Repeat the exercise at least three times. An alternative way of doing this exercise for those simply unable to stand or to grab hold of their foot in a standing position is to lie down (see below).

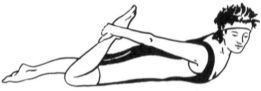

■ Stretching the outer thigh muscle

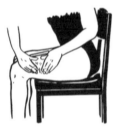

This exercise is particularly good for overcoming pain in the knees from tight muscles. Sitting on a chair first loosen the muscle up by gently squeezing it with your thumbs (see left). Now cross your legs with

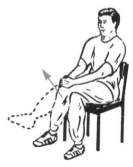

the leg you have been squeezing on top and holding the knee firmly with both hands pull it outwards (see right). You should feel the thigh of the leg on top stretching. Hold the stretch for ten seconds and release. Repeat three times. Change legs and do the same thing with the other leg.

Shiatsu for the thigh muscles

Applying finger pressure, or *shiatsu* in Japanese, to a series of points from where the thigh muscle meets the trunk down to the knee stimulates both circulation and nerve functioning. The area near the top of the leg is particularly important because this is the place where both the main artery and main nerve pass through. It is known as the inguinal region. Pressure should be applied by holding your thigh

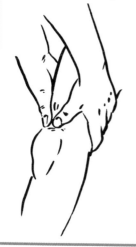

with your hands and using both thumbs, one on top of the other (see illustration left). Move methodically down each thigh, pressing firmly and evenly on each point for three seconds. Repeat three times.

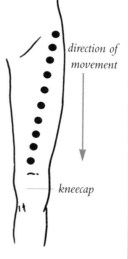

direction of movement

kneecap

■ Stretching the inner thigh muscles

Inner thigh weakness is common in people with leg problems from MS. Sit on the floor and, placing the soles of your feet together, pull your feet towards you so that you end up sitting as in the illustration right. Place your hands flat on your thighs close to your knees and press both legs

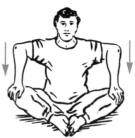

firmly and evenly downwards towards the floor. Hold this position for ten seconds and then release. Repeat three times. If you are wheel-chair-bound get help to sit on the floor and with the exercise itself.

Shiatsu for the inner thighs

Pressing on the points illustrated will also help the inner thigh muscles. This exercise encourages the drainage of lymph fluid from the legs and is particularly useful for those with leg pains and swollen ankles. With the leg turned outwards (as in the exercise on the previous page) apply pressure evenly, starting from the point where the leg joins the trunk and working methodically towards the knee (see right). Pressure should be applied for three seconds at every point. When you have finished repeat the exercise twice more.

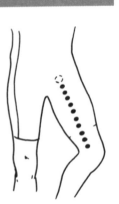

Strengthening exercises for legs and feet

After stretching exercises, which give mobility, the next most important step is to make sure muscles and sinews retain (or regain) their strength. The following exercises are all excellent for building up and strengthening the muscles and sinews of the legs and feet.

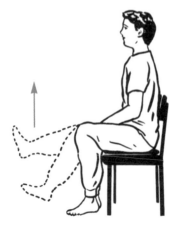

■ Strengthening the thigh muscle

Sit with your legs straight out. Tensing your thigh muscles, slowly straighten your knee, making sure it stays straight and with your toes bent towards you. Hold the position for ten seconds before lowering your leg. Repeat three times (see illustration left).

Once you get quite good you can make the exercise harder (and therefore better for you) by adding a weight to the leg to be lifted or a 'stretch band', a broad piece of rubber like a big elastic band obtainable from most sports and fitness centres.

Thigh and hip strengthening exercises from a sitting position

■ Hip strengthening

Sit as opposite, with both feet firmly on the floor but legs apart. Loop the stretch band around one thigh and ask your helper to hold both ends as in the illustration. Again keeping the other leg perfectly still and pointing forward pull against the band by trying to close your legs. All the pressure this time should be to the inside of your thigh.

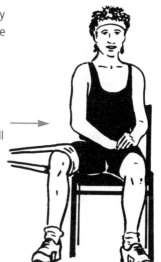

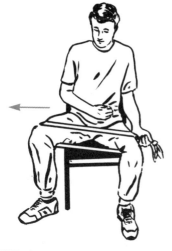

The illustration left shows you an alternative way to achieve the same result.

■ Thigh and upper leg strengthening

With your knees together tie a stretch band around your thighs just above the knees with enough looseness to let you move your knees about easily. Keeping one leg still move the other leg outwards as far as you can (see illustration below). It is important to keep both feet on the floor and not to swivel your hips to help the movement. Make your leg do all the work unaided.

This is an excellent exercise for people with problems of leg spasticity where the knees tend to knock together. The knees knock

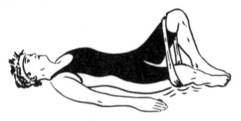

because the thigh muscles are too weak to keep them apart. That's why it's important when sitting normally to make a conscious effort to keep your knees apart and not to let them rest against each other. Letting them prop each other up only weakens them further because they are not doing any work.

■ Strengthening calf muscles

The following two exercises are excellent for helping control muscle spasms in the legs. Standing behind a chair or by a wall to steady yourself, raise yourself up and down using only your calf muscles. Make sure you keep a slight bend in the knees. Do ten 'lifts', rest for a short while and then do another set of ten twice more, resting in between. The exercise is more effective if you use a small sturdy box or brick to stand on (see left).

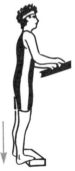

A harder variation on the above is, using the same sturdy box or brick, stand so that your foot is half off the step and your heel dropped below the level of the step (see right). Now lift yourself up using only your feet and calf muscles. Again, do the exercise in three sets of ten lifts, resting between each set.

Massage for the knees

The knee is the most complicated joint in the human body. It also takes more punishment than almost any other joint. It is small wonder, therefore, it can cause so much trouble and needs so much care and attention. Tiredness and fatigue is often felt first in the knees if the legs are under too much strain and this will cause them to become stiff and painful. Bending the knees can then become a problem. In people with MS painful knees is often the result of weak or tight thigh muscles. The following exercise can help enormously in this situation:

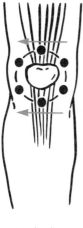

■ First, using your thumbs as described earlier in this chapter, apply pressure to the points shown in the diagram left around the area of the kneecap. This helps stimulate the release of the synovial fluid that keeps joints mobile.

■ Supporting your leg out straight massage the knee by placing both hands on the kneecap, one hand on top of the other, and using only light pressure make circular movements of the knee as in diagram right. Ten circles is enough.

■ Strengthening ankles

The following exercises are excellent for strengthening ankles and keeping them flexible:

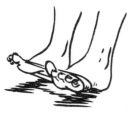

● Place an exercise or stretch band around both feet (preferably without any shoes or socks on, as illustration left) and, keeping your legs apart, force your toes outwards and upwards. Hold and release. Do this at least three to five times, depending on ankle strength.

● Sitting down, place a ball (a tennis ball is good) under one of your feet and roll it around on the floor applying as much downwards pressure as you can. Do the same thing with the other foot. This is a most envigorating exercise and many people experience an almost sensual tingling and 'aliveness' in their feet when they do it. What the exercise does is not just open 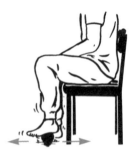 up the small bones of the feet but it stimulates the many reflex points on the feet linked to other parts of the body.

Massage and manipulation for legs and feet

Many people with MS suffer from muscle spasm. This is where the muscle becomes hard and tight and so loose their mobility and elasticity. The result can be an involuntary twitching of the muscles and this can happen at any time of the day or night. You put your feet up to relax or watch television and the next thing you know your legs are twitching and jerking uncontrollably. It can also happen after exercising. This is what is known as 'restless legs' and it can be a common feature of MS.

Muscle spasm can be caused by a buildup of lactic acid from lack of movement and exercise (though a poor diet and stress can also lead to lactic acid buildup) but, luckily, simple remedies are to hand – especially if you have someone to help you.

The most immediate remedy for restless legs, for example, is to get up and walk around for a while. Or you could do the stretching exercises in this chapter. Even if you are in bed and restless legs wake you up it is best to get up and walk around. This not only stretches the muscles but helps the acid disperse. If it is not possible for you to get out of bed try just stretching your leg out or get someone to help.

The next best step is to give your legs a good massage. If you cannot do this yourself for any reason get someone to do it for you. In fact even if you can do it yourself I would always advise trying to get someone to give you a massage. It is so much nicer and therefore usually more effective!

Start by massaging the back of the leg with long stroking movements, preferably using oil (see below). (The box 'Essential oils for

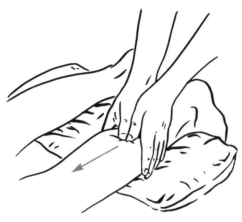

legs and feet' gives some suggestions for even greater benefit by adding the oils used in aromatherapy to your 'base' oil.) Make firm upward strokes the full length of the leg (but be careful to avoid too much downward pressure over the knee area and also never massage over varicose veins).

Next concentrate on the calf muscles. Calf muscles can contain a surprising amount of stress and massaging them can often be tender

but persevere – the tenderness will subside. Remember, always massage in an upward direction, towards the groin.

Make sure the muscles are warm before starting and use your thumbs in small, circular movements to

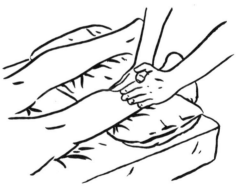

break down any knotted or hard tissue (see above).

You should stop immediately if for any reason the leg goes into spasm while you are massaging. Wait until the spasm has stopped and then work the toes of the foot backwards and forwards for a while before starting again. This first massage may not appear to help much at first but if you do it regularly enough you'll find it will get better and better. The effect of massage is cumulative.

Essential oils for legs and feet

To relax tense or hypertonic muscles
• Clary sage   • Jasmine
To improve muscle tone
• Juniper   • Rosemary   • Black pepper
My special tip
An excellent way for people with MS to use essential oils is in a foot-bath. About three or four drops of the chosen oil(s) in a bowl of warm water will do the job. This overcomes the problem not only of a bath being difficult for some people with MS to get into and out of again but the fact that a hot bath is not good for MS sufferers, tending to make the condition worse. Also the skin on the soles of the feet absorbs essential oils easily, so making it a very good way of getting the therapeutic properties of the oils into the body quickly.

An alternative to a footbath is to rub the oils into the feet in the normal way mixed with a neutral carrier oil.

■ Massage for feet

There are a separate set of routines for feet and they should not be overlooked. As the sections on reflexology in this book should make clear we ignore our feet at our cost. Keeping our feet flexible, for

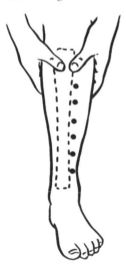

example, means we keep our spines flexible also. The following exercises will not only limber up the ankle but remove any stiffness and straighten the toes.

● Start by massaging or applying pressure, as you prefer, to the front part of the lower leg from the knee down to the ankle (see diagram left). This is the area of the important peroneal nerve and you may find it is quite tender. Pressing this area is also quite likely to make your foot move involuntarily. If this involuntary movement turns into a spasm stop, wait for the spasm to subside and continue. But don't continue until the spasm has subsided completely.

● Next, using your thumbs together in the shiatsu style described earlier, put pressure on the top of both feet on the points shown in the illustration below. This massages and stimulates all the tendons that work your toes. Apply the pressure on each point for up to a minute, depending on how tender each spot is. Try not to make it less than half a minute no matter how tender the spot.

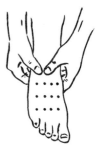

● Supporting the ankle with one hand, move all the toes backwards and forwards about ten times using the other hand. Do both feet this way.

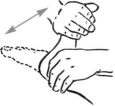

● Now rotate each foot ten times in one direction and ten times in the opposite direction. Massage the whole foot (preferably with oil) and continue the massage up the lower leg to the knee. This exercise is particularly good for helping with ankles that are puffy and stiff. Again, even if the ankles feel terribly inflexible and even painful at first persevere because they will loosen up and improve in time. If you find your legs swell, lifting them up as far as possible above chest height will help.

Reflexology for legs and feet

The diagrams opposite and on the next page show the various reflexology pressure points most helpful for legs and feet. A guide to treatment is on the next page also.

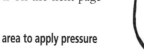 **area to apply pressure**

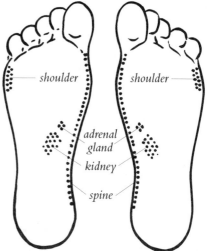

shoulder   shoulder

adrenal gland

kidney

spine

Reflexology points for weak legs and painful knees

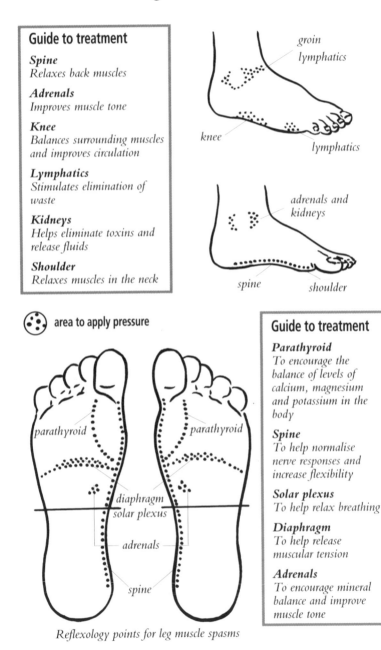

Guide to treatment

Spine
Relaxes back muscles

Adrenals
Improves muscle tone

Knee
Balances surrounding muscles
and improves circulation

Lymphatics
Stimulates elimination of
waste

Kidneys
Helps eliminate toxins and
release fluids

Shoulder
Relaxes muscles in the neck

groin
lymphatics

knee

lymphatics

adrenals and
kidneys

spine   shoulder

● area to apply pressure

parathyroid   parathyroid

diaphragm
solar plexus

adrenals

spine

Guide to treatment

Parathyroid
To encourage the
balance of levels of
calcium, magnesium
and potassium in the
body

Spine
To help normalise
nerve responses and
increase flexibility

Solar plexus
To help relax breathing

Diaphragm
To help release
muscular tension

Adrenals
To encourage mineral
balance and improve
muscle tone

Reflexology points for leg muscle spasms

▦ Dietary and nutritional support for legs and feet

Problems with legs and feet such as muscle spasms, muscle tremors and foot cramps can be caused by an imbalance of calcium and magnesium while a potassium deficiency can cause muscle weakness. Hair analysis reports frequently reveal that magnesium and calcium levels are out of balance in people with MS and that potassium levels are low.

Potassium is involved in helping transmit nerve impulses to muscles and in activating the digestive enzymes that convert food into energy while magnesium is vital for the correct working of the muscles and the nervous system. Apart from muscle spasms, tremors and cramps, symptoms of magnesium deficiency are depression, poor memory, irritability and similar nervous disorders.

The good news is that problems in any of these areas can sometimes be put right quite easily by simply adjusting your diet.

Nutritional deficiencies, though, are not only the result of not taking in enough of the right nutrients in your daily diet but can also be caused by a problem the body has in absorbing nutrients properly, usually because of a lack of hydrochloric acid in the stomach or the right level of pancreatic enzymes.

The solution for magnesium deficiency this way is an alkaline diet supplemented with 400iu (international units) of vitamin E every day. A good alkaline diet is 70 per cent 'water content' foods such as fruit, vegetables, wholegrain nuts and yoghurt and 30 per cent foods such as fish, liver, chicken, eggs and cheese. Tea and coffee should be limited.

I have found that improving the digestion of people with MS by prescribing digestive enzymes can help muscle spasm dramatically. If you want advice on taking digestive enzymes – and I recommend you do – it is best to consult a qualified nutritional therapist. (See Appendix B 'The "leaky gut" syndrome' and 'Taking Supplements'.)

Fruit, vegetables and wholegrains are also good for boosting potassium levels but potassium can be taken as a food supplement as well.

Where deficiency is the result of a lack of digestive enzymes, supplementation with enzymes and regular abdominal massage often produces excellent results.

Dealing with pain in the legs and feet

■ Leg pain

General pain in the legs and any other form of altered sensation can be due to tight muscles in the lower back. So, once more, you need to look to the back as well as the legs for the solution. Back exercises such as 'The Cat' stretch and side-bends (see chapter 6) will improve muscle mobility and alleviate some symptoms.

■ Legs giving way

Many people with leg weakness as a result of MS, myself included, suffer from the unnerving experience of one or other of their legs (and sometimes both together) giving way under them for no obvious reason. The causes can be many but the main ones – apart from the obvious of poor nerve transmission due to MS – are:

● a weakness in the knee joint(s)
● a bruised nerve in the back
● poor posture
● walking badly.

Something as apparently simple as walking badly or poor posture (the two are obviously connected anyway) can cause the legs in anyone to give way suddenly but it is far more likely in someone whose leg movement is already affected by MS.

What happens is that the muscular imbalance caused by the poor walking or posture can put a knee or hip joint under such stress and strain that the body's automatic response is to want to rest that joint. Letting the leg give way is a normal reaction of the body to protect a joint under stress.

The solution is long-term and involves trying to realign your spine into a correct posture, learning to walk properly and strengthening the muscles of both the back and legs to protect the various joints affected. It is important to remember not to try to force the pace by putting unnecessary pressure on muscles, bones and tissues in these areas. Treatment must be gentle and improvement gradual. Patience is vital.

Another tip is to slow your walking down and walk correctly heel-to-toe, so eventually re-educating yourself to walk properly again.

◾ Knee pain

An MS patient of mine once came to see me complaining of pain in the left knee that she had been suffering from for some weeks. The exercise routine I had given her for her MS had helped but the pain was still there. Because she obviously put less weight on the painful knee, she walked in a lop-sided manner and this, I soon discovered after examining her again, was the cause of the problem.

Muscular spasm in the lower back had caused her to develop a tilt-ed pelvis and altered the way her thighs muscles were working on her kneecap. This, in turn, was putting undue strain on her knee joint and this was the cause of the pain. In other words, the source of her problem was her lower back muscles, not the knee itself.

I recommended rest, localised heat treatment (using a hot-water bottle), stretching (see page 116), and light exercises to correct the working of the thigh muscles. I also prescribed an elasticated knee support and, because the condition was not too severe, advised her to see her doctor for anti-inflammatory medication and/or ultrasound treatment. For her back pain, we gave her massage, ultra-sound, faradic treatment and stretching exercises to help relieve the spasm.

Knee pain can also be the result of weak thigh and calf muscles. If this is the case with you carrying out the exercises on pages 120-122 will help. If you don't know or are not sure if you have weak leg muscles see a physical therapist, physiotherapist or other qualified person such as a fitness instructor who can advise you.

◾ Ankle pain

Another patient, Julie, came to see me with pain in her left ankle whenever she pointed her toe or bent over and stretched. She complained that it always happened when she was making the bed for example.

Examination showed she had a very tender achilles tendon and there was obvious swelling between the tendon and heel bone. In her case I advised wearing open back shoes to relieve the pressure, light exercises such as ankle turns (see page 100) and, again, anti-inflammatory medication and/or ultrasound. An alternative to open back shoes is to put a foam rubber ring (like a large corn plaster) into the back of the shoe.

In general, both ill-fitting shoes and a dragging foot can cause problems with the feet and obviously the last is more common in MS. If you drag your foot and do not make a conscious effort to correct the problem – by walking more slowly and picking the foot up and putting it down correctly without dragging it, for example – you are quite likely to suffer from muscle pain and weakness. But with a little thought and effort the problem can be helped.

sexual health

The following three chapters all deal with problems resulting from MS that are not really specific to any one particular part of the body – though sexual problems clearly involve mainly the sexual organs – and do not necessarily have direct physical causes.

For example, a sexual problem such as impotence is obviously a physical symptom but it can just as easily be the result of feeling tired and depressed as having MS. In that sense it is not at all specific to people with MS. Impotence is a problem common to many men.

Although each of the following chapters deals with sexual problems, tiredness and depression separately, in reality they are closely linked. Depression can lead to tiredness that can lead to sexual problems, and sexual problems can lead to depression that can lead to tiredness, and so on.

So it is a good idea to read all three chapters as if they are part of the same problem. And indeed, you will find many of the treatments I recommend in all three chapters are the same also.

But though it is true that mental and emotional problems that any-one can experience can cause sexual problems – it can be caused by work or money problems, for example – it is also true that sexual problems in MS can be the result of causes that are specific to MS.

Physical causes of sexual problems in women with MS are commonly lack of vaginal lubrication and sensation, muscle spasm and poor bladder control coupled with decreased ability to have an orgasm, while in men the problem is mainly an inability to have an erection (impotence) or ejaculate also leading to reduced orgasm experience.

Drugs given for MS can also be to blame. Some tranquillisers and antidepressants can depress sexual response, for example, as can tobacco, cannabis, cocaine and too much alcohol. Other physical causes of what doctors call sexual 'dysfunction', particularly of impotence in men, is heart disease, diabetes, having mumps as an adult and anti-ulcer drugs.

Having MS is no reason whatsoever to stop or limit sexual activity if you don't want to and, fortunately, a wide variety of treatments is available that can be very effective for both men and women in helping to maintain both the desire and the means. Covering psychological as well as physical needs, these include counselling and psychotherapy, massage with aromatherapy oils, reflexology, nutritional therapy (diet and supplements) and exercise.

General treatments for lack of sexual desire and impotence

Whatever the underlying reasons for the problem you are experiencing the first need for anyone worried about reduced sexual response is to talk about it. Talking about it – communicating your anxieties and concerns – is very definitely the first step to solving it. Obviously your partner is the best person to talk to if you can since he or she is the person most affected and the closest to you.

But if this is not possible for any reason – and sexual problems are often some of the hardest for coupes to share – then my advice is to seek out a sympathetic and understanding friend. I think this is better than the standard advice to see your family doctor. Of course if you are confident in your doctor then there is no problem. And sometimes you may well need the advice of someone with specialist medical knowledge.

Most of the time a doctor will probably refer you to a trained counsellor, psychotherapist or even sex therapist anyway and seeing a specialist in listening to problems and suggesting solutions is also an excellent option, especially one experienced in the sex problems of people with MS.

Since stress and anxiety can be one of the biggest causes of sexual problems this one step alone can work wonders as it can help to remove the underlying tension they can produce. Many therapists won't just stop at talking, though. They are quite likely to suggest other approaches to help you relax and feel more at peace with yourself as well as, at the same time, reawaken your needs and desires.

Good advice for anyone, man or woman, wanting to improve their sexual health is

- eat a good balanced diet
- do regular exercise
- cut out smoking
- don't drink too much alcohol.

In addition I would recommend the following, particularly for those with MS:

- massage with essential oils *(aromatherapy)*
- reflexology
- nutritional therapy
- special exercises.

Massage with essential oils

Teaching yourself and your partner to communicate physically as well as mentally and verbally is quite one of the most effective ways of helping overcome any form of sexual problem, whether you have MS or not. And probably the best way to communicate physically is to massage one another. Better still, massage one another with essential oils. Believe me, it works wonders!

Oils said to be best for sexual problems are rose, neroli (orange flower), ylang ylang, jasmine and sandalwood. See the following chart for guidance on how best to use these oils but remember the general rule not to mix them and use only a few drops in a neutral base oil (grapeseed oil is good).

Essential oils for sexual health

Oils	Action	Best for
Rose	Relaxant, antidepressant, aphrodisiac	*Lack of sexual desire, PMS, regulating menstruation*
Neroli	Relaxant, aphrodisiac	*Lack of desire and impotence*
Ylang Ylang	Relaxant, aphrodisiac	*Lack of desire and impotence*
Jasmine	Relaxant, sedative, calming, antidepressant	*Lack of desire and impotence*
Sandalwood	Relaxant, sedative, calming	*Lack of desire*

Reflexology

Massaging and putting pressure on the areas on the feet shown in the diagram below will help problems of a physical sexual nature in both men and women.

● area to apply pressure

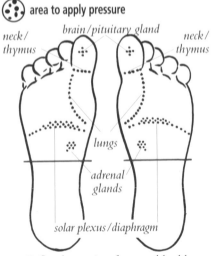

neck/thymus   brain/pituitary gland   neck/thymus

lungs

adrenal glands

solar plexus/diaphragm

Reflexology points for sexual health

Guide to treatment

Pituitary gland
Regulates hormone production

Neck/thyroid
Relaxes and balances energy levels, produces hormones for development of nervous system

Lungs
Regulates breathing

Solar/plexus/diaphragm
Relaxes breathing

Brain
Soothes nerves for better sexual response

Adrenal glands
Revitalises the body

Ovaries/testes/fallopian tubes
Improves circulation to sexual organs

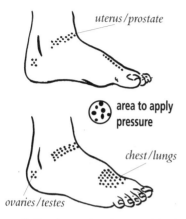

uterus/prostate

area to apply pressure

chest/lungs

ovaries/testes

Reflexology points for sexual health

For example, pressure on the pituitary gland on the big toe is said to stimulate the production of the sex hormones. The effect is not to arouse you sexually, as some essential oils can do, but more to promote the right conditions for sex by relaxing and calming and increasing the communication between two people. As described earlier, apply the pressure evenly for at least five seconds.

Diet and nutrition

Diet and exercise are two of the most effective ways of stimulating your body to respond sexually – mainly because they are both vital for overall health and vitality. And in an adult a healthy and vital body is a sexual body. So make sure you not only keep active by exercising (see the next section) but by eating properly. That means not only eating a balanced diet but, for sexual problems, foods that are good for the sexual or reproductive system.

Fortunately foods that are good for the reproductive system in adults are also very tasty so there is no real excuse for avoiding this part of the programme. In fact most people find it very enjoyable! For example, three of the most important nutrients for the reproductive system are the vitamins C and E and the mineral zinc (particularly important for men). The list below shows you the many good food sources:

■ Zinc

Meat/seafood	Lamb, pork, chicken, oysters, clams, prawns
Vegetables	Carrots, beans, parsley, potatoes, garlic
Nuts and seeds	Almonds, walnuts and pumpkin seeds

■ Vitamin C

Fruit	All citrus fruits, berries, rosehips, kiwifruits, cherries
Vegetables	All green and leafy vegetables, potatoes, tomatoes

■ Vitamin E

Vegetables   Broccoli, brussel sprouts, spinach, vegetable oils
Nuts & cereals Most nuts and seeds, wheatgerm, wholemeal grains.

Don't worry if you eat little of the above foods, though, or don't like any of them. It's possible to get the same level of nutrients, or higher, by taking food supplements, either as tablets or powders. In fact in today's world many people don't get enough of the right nutrients just by eating a balanced diet and so it is almost essential in many cases they take food supplements to boost their daily intake. This is particularly so if they need more than the average amount to help support an unbalanced system.

The table below shows you the right amounts of zinc, vitamins C and E and other nutrients to take to supplement your daily diet if you have sexual problems. But rather than just assume a deficiency I would always recommend having a hair mineral analysis done first. This will not only show up a lack of the right nutrients but also if you have picked up too many of the wrong things such as lead, mercury and other toxic heavy metals (usually from the environment).

Food supplements for sexual health

Nutrient	Daily dose	Action
MEN		
Zinc	15mg	*Supports prostate gland and sex organs*
Vitamin C	1000mg	*Improves sperm quality and mobility*
Vitamin E	400iu*	*Increases fertility and restores potency*
L-Arginine	500mg	*Increases sperm count*
WOMEN		
Zinc	15mg	*Supports reproductive organs*
Vitamin C	1000mg	*Supports repair and growth of tissue cells*
Vitamin E	400iu*	*Increases fertility, strengthens cells and slows the ageing process.*

* Start with 200iu and increase gradually to the recommended dose. Not to be taken if using blood-thinning drugs such as heparin and warfarin.

Other natural remedies

Though not strictly foods so much as herbal medicines, two other supplements are said to be good for sexual problems and you can find these in most good health stores. They are ginseng/Siberian ginseng and ginkgo biloba.

■ Ginseng

A favourite remedy for sexual problems in China, ginseng is claimed to relax someone who is tense but stimulate a tired person. It is also said to increase the efficiency of the nerve impulses, improving mental performance and memory, as well as increase the activity of white blood cells (essential for the proper working of the immune system remember). Other functions supposed to be helped include appetite and digestion. Most significant of all, though, it has the reputation of being able to improve stamina and enhance sexual performance for both men and women.

■ Ginkgo biloba

Another ancient Chinese remedy (in fact ginkgo biloba is the oldest tree on Earth, a relic of the days when dinosaurs walked the planet!), extract of ginkgo biloba has proved so successful at treating some cases of impotence that drugs companies are now busy trying to synthesise the active compounds at work in the plant so that they can patent a drug based on it. To make doubly sure they will make a fortune they are also trying to ban its sale in its natural form. Public beware!

Ginkgo compounds (known as *bioflavonoids*) also have the ability to maintain the circulation of the blood to the brain (so helping with memory and concentration) as well as to the body's extremities, such as hands and feet.

Physical therapy/Massage

Both men and women can be helped by manipulation and massage of the lower part of the back where many sexual problems have their physical source. Symptoms can be low back pain or ache accompanied by tight muscles or muscles in spasm. All these things not only affect sexual response and performance but are a sign of impaired sexual response.

Manipulation of the back by a skilled physical therapist – especially using techniques that stretch the muscles of the spine and the tissues attached to it – or massage by someone equally skilled, perhaps using one or more of the essential oils listed on page 136, is an excellent way to ease the tension and ache in the lower back as well as promote a return to proper, or at least better, sexual function.

For more details turn to chapter 6 on back problems in MS.

Rebounding for more vitality

Regular use of a mini-trampoline – also known as 'rebounding' – is an excellent way to improve vitality. Bouncing up and down on a rebounder not only exercises the heart – and a healthy heart is crucial in the battle for more energy for anyone – but encourages the circulation of fluids, particularly those of the all-important lymph system (see chapter 2). More energy usually means more interest in activity of all sorts, including sex. So a mini-trampoline or 'rebounder' is an excellent investment.

You can use a mini-trampoline even if your balance is affected by getting someone reliable to hold one hand or arm while you bounce as in the illustration opposite. Alternatively, if you are wheelchair-bound, you can sit on the side of the rebounder and ask someone to hold you while another person bounces up and down. The effect of them bouncing and you sitting is to make you bounce too - and so you get all the benefits without having to make the effort! I love it!

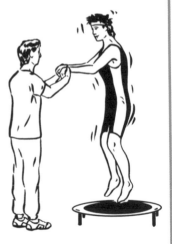

tiredness and fatigue

Tiredness and fatigue is another very common problem in MS but in many ways it is one of the hardest to deal with because it is invisible. You may look well to other people – who may even say things like 'Oh, you're looking well' – but only you know how desperately tired and worn-out you really feel inside. And unlike most physical symptoms you can get help with, 'MS fatigue' is a symptom you have to deal with on your own.

I say 'MS fatigue' deliberately because the sort of fatigue experienced by people with MS is quite different from normal fatigue, and certainly very different from the fatigue an athlete, say, may feel after running a marathon. Most people recover quite quickly from fatigue as the result of deliberate exertion or exercise simply by resting. But the fatigue associated with MS is where everything seems to be a problem all the time. Even the simplest of tasks can feel like trying to climb a mountain and no amount of rest seems to make any difference. You still feel like someone has wrung you out and hung you up to dry!

The reason is that MS fatigue is not just physical. It can be mental and emotional as well, and as anyone knows who has experienced either mental and emotional tiredness can often be far more draining than physical tiredness – as well as much harder to identify and do something about. To complicate matters further, all three causes are frequently interlinked, so that physical tiredness can cause mental and emotional fatigue and vice versa.

I remember my own experience vividly. The worst period was in 1988. I was tired for no obvious reason and depressed the whole time, crying at the drop of a hat at the slightest thing. My husband would come home and find me crying and ask me why and I couldn't tell him. I really had absolutely no idea what the matter was.

It was quite the most awful period of my life. Getting out of bed in the morning would be a huge effort and when I did manage to struggle up I felt as if I had not slept for a week and been run over by a bus at the same time. I would have a shower and then have to lie on the bathroom floor for literally half an hour before I could move. If I wanted to wash my hair it had to wait for the next day because I simply could not do the two things in the same day. Every time I tried to do anything I would feel so bad that I ended up doing nothing. Day after day, from morning to night, I would just watch television. My husband did many of the household chores for me because I couldn't. I never went out and became ever more weak and depressed. It was truly a nightmare – a nightmare I know is shared by many people with MS.

It took me many years to understand my problem and learn how to handle the peculiar fatigue experienced by people with MS. But the result is that I feel I am now in a position to pass on my knowledge to others so that they no longer have to suffer as I did.

Symptoms and causes of MS fatigue

Classic symptoms of fatigue are dark circles under the eyes (often from lack of proper sleep and rest), headaches, listlessness, lethargy, pains in the muscles and joints, insomnia and depression. Harder to pin down, because everyone is so different, are precise causes. They can be physical or psychological or, more usually, a combination of both.

An example of a purely physical cause of fatigue is low blood sugar (hypoglycaemia). Others are sensitivity to or intolerance of certain foods (generally known as 'food allergy'), vegan dieting, overgrowth of the yeast *candida albicans* in the gut, hormonal imbalance (a cause of pre-menstrual syndrome), iron-deficiency anaemia (a common cause of tiredness, particularly in menstruating women - though iron deficiency can also be caused by a lack of vitamin B12), heavy periods and pregnancy. But tiredness and fatigue can also be caused by depression (see chapter 11 for more on dealing with depression).

Two good examples of how varied fatigue can be in MS are the cases of Alison and Alan.

Alison had many of the classic symptoms of MS when she came to see me in September 1992. She had been officially diagnosed two years before with tingling in the fingers and toes, night cramps, tender calf muscles and general muscle weakness, loss of appetite, constipation, insomnia – and constant fatigue.

Apart from glandular fever as a child, Alison had had no other serious illnesses – but she had suffered a whiplash injury in a car accident five years before coming to see me and had then tragically lost her daughter in another car crash two years later. Alison's health suffered seriously as a result of these events and she began having problems eating. Her first MS-like symptoms – tingling and numbness – started soon after.

I soon discovered that not only did Alison have the tight spasms in her back I find in so many people with MS but her diet was poor. She was verging on the under-nourished by not eating much and she was also drinking huge amounts of coffee with sugar: about 15 mugs a day, she said! I recommended a change in diet and physical therapy.

Alison found both quite difficult, particularly the removal of caffeine and sugar from her diet. This had to be done gradually because of the withdrawal symptoms common in people who take in large amounts of these chemicals. Both can increase energy levels in the short-term but over the long-term they promote depression, headache, mood swings – and fatigue. Fatigue is also a symptom of caffeine withdrawal, which is why many people can get into a vicious downward spiral of fatigue: they drink coffee to stop themselves feeling tired, but they feel more tired when the effect wears off, and so drink more coffee, and feel more tired, and so on...

It took Alison six weeks of hard work to break her cycle but she finally managed it – with a little nagging from me! We also gave her some manipulation which she found uncomfortable, including soft tissue work on her spine. The most immediate benefit she experienced was improvement in bladder control and she also became less constipated. Finally, after about two months, the feeling returned to her hands and the tingling stopped.

Alan started on my programme in September 1994. He had been diagnosed with MS in 1989 even though his symptoms were slight – consisting mainly of lack of sensation in his nerve endings, fatigue, sluggishness and poor concentration. Then aged 32 he had suffered from asthma throughout his life and the asthma was far more disabling than the MS. Walking even small distances made him tired and breathless.

Alan had been divorced four years previously and lived on his own. At work he sat in front of a computer all day and when I saw him he was overweight and had dark circles under his eyes. The first thing I did was go through his diet and found that he ate not just badly but terribly! He hardly ever had breakfast, had usually just a cheese sandwich for lunch, and either fish and chips or omelette and chips for supper. He was also a chocoholic, drinking around two pints of hot chocolate with milk a day. I felt sure at once that many of his symptoms were due more to his appalling diet than MS.

I asked Alan to avoid all dairy products and chocolate – and within 48 hours the dark circles under his eyes had begun to disappear. After a few weeks the general aches and pains he had complained of before improved and he became obviously more alert, cheerful and interested in the world around him. He did not lose much weight but he was clearly getting the right nutrients.

Alan still has his minor MS symptoms but the changes to his diet and lifestyle alone have proved enough, in his case, to help not only his asthma but to relieve all his symptoms of fatigue, sluggishness and poor concentration.

■ Treatment

As the stories of Alison and Alan make clear, my recommended treatment for MS fatigue falls into three main areas:

- Diet and nutrition (this is the most important)
- Massage, including aromatherapy and reflexology
- Manipulation and exercises.

Diet and nutrition

As a general rule I have found there is no doubt that the worse some-one's diet the more likely they are to feel tired, whether they have MS or not. Junk food and eating large amounts of sugar can cause fatigue and a 'tired-all-the-time' feeling in almost anyone by creatings swings of high and low in the levels of sugar in the blood.

Carole is another good example of someone with MS with severe fatigue who I found I could help enormously simply by suggesting a change in diet to improve her nutritional intake. Carole ran a pub and found not only that she could no longer work the hours she used to, even with MS, but that she was also liable to be short-tempered and to suffer from extreme swings in mood.

When she told me her typical eating day I knew the reason at once. Starting at 8am, she would have a breakfast of coffee and a cigarette, followed by a lunch of an alcoholic drink and a cigarette, and end the day with a bar snack – and a cigarette. In between she would smoke more cigarettes.

I considered Carole's problem was mainly one of low blood sugar rather than MS. A hair mineral analysis showed she was also deficient in a range of essential nutrients and so I started her on a programme of better diet and nutritional supplements. The improvement was dramatic. Within a short time, Carole was back to working her long hours with hardly any problems of fatigue at all – and, as important, hardly any symptoms of MS either.

For me, the link between diet and MS for many people is now beyond doubt. This had been confirmed for me long ago when I found that one of the most effective dietary treatments for MS fatigue is the system known as 'food combining'. I had tried all the different diets in my effort to improve my condition, but it was the 'food com-bining diet' that I found gave me the most energy. On it I felt really well and not deprived of anything.

Food combining and the 'Hay Diet'

Excessive tiredness after eating a meal is a problem I come across often in people with MS. I also find that hot food is almost certain to cause fatigue in someone already weak for whatever reason, not just MS.

In both cases the treatment I find most helpful is to separate protein and carbohydrates when eating. Generally speaking this means not eating, for example, meat, fish and cheese (protein) with potatoes, bread or flour (carbohydrates).

An American doctor, Howard Hay, first discovered the problems caused by combining protein and carbohydrates in the 1930s and this principle is now known as the Hay principle of food combining or, more usually, just 'The Hay Diet'. What happens is that combining meat and potatoes in the same meal, for example, makes the body work twice as hard to break down (or 'metabolize') these foods when they are both in the digestive system at the same time. The energy that should be going into your bloodstream for the rest of your body is going into helping out your digestive system instead. This, in turn, contributes to tiredness. So the answer here is to have meat with vegetables but no potatoes. Or pasta and vegetables or salad together but no fish or cheese.

I have found that people who stick to this way of eating feel nothing like so tired after a meal and have more energy. Try it and see. Following the tips in the box below will also help.

8 steps for sustained energy

1 Always have breakfast, no matter how little

2 Drink plenty of clean (ie filtered or bottled) water – ideally, at least 1.5 to two litres a day.

3 Eat at least five portions of fresh fruit and vegetables a day.

4 Eat at least three meals a week using vegetable sources of protein such as tofu, pulses and nuts.

5 Eat complex carbohydrates such as wholemeal pasta rather than refined simple carbohydrates such as biscuits, sweets and white bread.

6 Avoid all stimulants such as coffee, tea, alcohol and nicotine (tobacco).

7 Always chew your food well and try not to eat in a hurry.

8 Never over-eat.

Note: Eating in a hurry and over-eating can slow you down more than anything else.

Food supplementation

Feeling tired for no obvious physical or emotional reason may be due to a poor diet or a lack of basic nutrients in the body or both. In other words, your general diet may be excellent but you can still be lacking in certain vitamins and minerals for reasons that are specific to the way your body is working (or not working). That's where taking extra nutrients, particularly minerals, as 'food supplements' can be helpful. Supplements for fatigue are summarised in the box 'Food supplements for fatigue' below.

Food supplements for fatigue

Nutrient	Daily dose
Vitamin B complex	50mg
Vitamin C	1-2g
Co-enzyme Q10	up to 30mg
Zinc	15mg
Iron (avoid sulphate forms)	28mg
Magnesium	200-400mg
Chromium GTF	100mcg
Ginseng	600mg

Massage

Massage has a powerfully relaxing effect on the human body. But the wonderful thing about it is that it is the sort of relaxation that, done properly, does not make you feel wiped out afterwards (though it can if you are under excessive tension and strain at the time), but revitalises and revivifies. So massage is effective for MS fatigue because it gives the body time to unwind, as it were, and rewind more efficiently. As always, the two types of massage I particularly recommend for MS, including MS fatigue, are aromatherapy and reflexology.

Aromatherapy

The oils that help with fatigue are all stimulants and if you read what I've said above you'll see this is not as strange as it may seem. The combined effect of massage, which relaxes, with oils that stimulate promotes the 'unwinding-rewinding properly' process I describe exactly. Note that the word 'stimulate' here does not mean the same as when talking about coffee, tea, alcohol or other drugs. Those are stimulants that lift you up high and fast but drop you down just as far and fast afterwards – leaving you no better off and usually a lot worse because they have a 'burn-out' effect. Essential oils that stimulate are not stimulants but stimulating: their effect is more gradual and subtle but longer-lasting.

Important note Massage with relaxing oils can have the adverse effect on someone with MS by making them too relaxed. An example is a particular patient of mine, Kay, who went to a health farm where the aromatherapist used 'sedating' oils, as she described them, because she, like so many others,

> **Stimulating oils to use for MS fatigue are:**
>
> *For physical fatigue*
> Basil, nutmeg, thyme, geranium, rosemary and marjoram
>
> *For mental fatigue*
> Rosemary, nutmeg

believed that they would 'calm and relax' the nervous system and that this must be good for someone with MS. In fact it has the opposite effect by making the nervous system so relaxed it makes symptoms worse and thereby increases anxiety and depression. It took Kay nearly four days to recover from her experience and so always be careful not to use relaxing oils of any great strength in cases of MS.

Another important point to make here is not to let the use of essential oils become a substitute for proper rest. Don't use them, in other words, as you might tea or coffee to allow you to go on working at the same unhealthy pace as if they were a 'quick fix' drug. You will do nothing to overcome constant tiredness if you use essential oils this way. Always aim to get enough rest and a good night's sleep to allow the body to replenish energy naturally.

Essential oils can help here too and the ones to use, especially to ensure a sound night's sleep, are lavender and chamomile. Both have a calming and soothing effect and are especially good if placed on the pillow at bedtime.

■ Reflexology

Reflexology is another of the key therapies in successfully overcoming MS fatigue. Reflexology helps the body to relax and a relaxed body helps to heal itself. The areas to concentrate are shown in the diagram below.

Guide to treatment

Diaphragm
To relax

Heart
To improve circulation

Thymus
To help balance metabolism

Brain
To balance the central nervous system

Pituitary gland
To balance hormone levels

Spine
To relax and regulate nerve impulses

Pancreas
To balance blood sugar levels (improves energy)

Liver
To release energy (glucose) into bloodstream

Adrenal glands
To stimulate hormone release and regulate stress response

My special tip To stimulate and enliven the whole body stamp your foot on the ground or get someone to lightly hit the soles of your feet with a book or something of a similar weight.

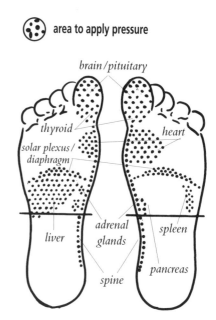

● area to apply pressure

Reflexology points for tiredness and fatigue

Treatment for psychological causes of MS

This book does not concentrate too heavily on psychological treatments because it is not really my speciality. But I have looked into the situation and in my experience some of the most effective treatments for psychological (mental and emotional) causes of 'MS fatigue' involve the use of:

- visualisation
- yoga.

The best information on this for people with MS is contained in Meir Schneider's book *The Handbook of Self-Healing* and Howard Kent's *Yoga for the Disabled* (see Appendices C and D for more details) but the following very brief summaries give you some idea of the approaches they recommend.

Visualization

According to Meir Schneider, an American who effectively cured himself of blindness and now runs a school of self-healing in San Francisco, when an area of the body suffers from lack of sensation, mobility or normal function – as in MS – the mind can all too easily 'disengage' from the area affected. It decides that area is ineffective and useless and so writes it off as redundant.

Visualization is a way of preventing the mind losing interest and making sure it continues to send messages and signals along the nerves to the affected part. It does this by making use of the power of the imagination. Visualization is simply using the imagination to influence the body.

In a way it is a bit like day-dreaming but instead of aimless, random thoughts and pictures of the sort most of us have when we day-dream, visualization is the art of creating deliberately directed thoughts and pictures for a specific purpose. Imagining sheep jumping over a fence to get to sleep or sunbathing by a warm, calm, blue sea to relax is exactly the process.

Visualization is a way of forming a bridge between the body and the mind and is one of the most powerful – and still most under-estimated and least understood – tools for healing we have. In MS it can be used not only to encourage nerve signals to be directed properly to physically affected parts of the body but also to overcome psychological symptoms of fatigue and depression.

To help problems with legs, for example, you could imagine signals shooting at full strength from the brain, down the spinal cord and along the nerve fibres to the legs and the legs working as you know they should. You may decide to see this a bit like they sometimes show it in cartoons or adverts on television – as a blaze of white light shooting along like a train through a tunnel or as a racing car roaring along a race-track.

In other words, imagine whatever you need to achieve the result you want using whatever images you find most helpful and effective. To relax, imagine something you find most relaxing; to feel more energetic, imagine something that makes you feel you have more energy; to feel sexier imagine something that makes you feel sexy, and so on. It can be fun as well as easy, and it really does work if you persevere.

For further information on Meir Schneider's self-healing approach see Appendix C: Resources.

■ Yoga

Everyone has heard of yoga but not many people realize that it is actually a major part of a complete system of healing evolved centuries ago in India known as Ayurveda or 'Science of Life'. Yoga, which means 'union', is not just movement and exercises – though that is what it is best known for – but also a way of learning how to breathe correctly and use the mind to heal. So it is a system that, done properly, looks after the body, mind and emotions all at once.

Learning the right exercises to tackle specific symptoms of MS is best not done on your own. It really needs the guidance of someone who knows what they are doing. The pioneer of the effective use of yoga in MS is the British therapist Howard Kent and I recommend anyone who is interested in learning how to use yoga to help with their particular symptoms to contact the Yoga for Health Foundation which he founded and still runs. The foundation is also the only distributor now of Howard's excellent little book *Yoga for the Disabled (see Appendix C)*.

See also chapter 11.

depression

Depression is another of those problems very common in MS that is not limited to people with MS. Everyone suffers from depression at some stage in their lives, just as they do colds and flu. In fact it was been well described as 'the common cold of mental and emotional disorders.' But clearly people with MS have a more than average reason for feeling low and the chances are that the times when it gets the better of them will happen more often than most. So what to do about it?

The first thing is to understand a bit about it. Depression is not simply feeling sad, 'woolly-headed' or 'not quite with it' as some peope with MS have described it to me. As well as symptoms of anxiety, tiredness, lethargy and despair, depression can show itself in much less obvious ways. Insomnia, early morning waking, changes in eating habits such as eating too much or too little, indigestion, constipation, headaches, pains in different parts of the body, and prob-lems with concentration and memory can all be due to depression.

Other symptoms are dry and lack-lustre skin and hair, high blood pressure, lack of interest in sex, irritability, temperamental outbursts, and a whole range of feelings reflecting negative self-worth: 'I'm worth nothing, no one loves me or needs me, I'm useless, stupid, hopeless, it's all my fault, I'm to blame'...the list is endless.

The causes of depression are as wide and varied as the symptoms and range from the seemingly psychological to the much less obvious physical. For example, you may think you are depressed because of your MS and that would be a quite natural thing to think. But depression can be caused by a basic nutritional deficiency as much as by feeling unloved and helpless. Other purely physical causes of depression can be hormonal imbalances (particularly in women), an underactive thyroid gland (hypothyroidism), and heart disease.

Sometimes simply improving your diet and taking extra food supplements to correct the chemical imbalances in your body can work wonders on their own. For example, a 'woolly' feeling accompanied by tiredness can be due to a magnesium deficiency. Stress, anxiety and 'acid stomach' can all cause the body to excrete large amounts of magnesium and these need to be replaced. Replacement can cause the problem to subside and even disappear altogether sometimes. At other times, the services of a sympathetic physical therapist, aromatherapist or reflexologist can make the necessary difference.

The point is that depression is usually manageable and you don't have to swallow a fistful of drugs from the doctor to do it. In fact the more you can keep away from strong synthetic drugs altogether the better, for whatever condition.

I know – I've been there and come back!

Treatments

Since the mind and body are closely interlinked, the best treatment for depression in MS, whether purely psychological or definitely physical, is a mixture of both physical and psychological therapy. For MS I usually recommend a combination of

- diet and nutrition
- massage and romatherapy
- reflexology
- counselling.

The counselling is the easy bit so let me deal with that first.

◼ Counselling

'Counselling' always sounds a bit grand to me. It's really about talking – and that's something I'm told I do quite well. So what I mean when I say counselling is having a good old-fashioned chat about anything and everything: problems, fears, past disappointments, future expectations and so on.

Many people with MS who come to see me are depressed. If they don't tell me they are I can soon see they are. It is written all over them. They have either just been diagnosed with MS or have livedwith it for many years and are just plain miserable and upset. What it usually comes down to is the fact that they cannot accept they have MS and so cannot come to terms with it. But coming to terms with MS is one of the first and most important things to do with it.

This does not mean giving in to it. Quite the opposite, in fact. It means saying, 'okay, so I have MS – so what? It's only a name. But I've got it and now I'm going to start doing something about it. I'm going to start living for a start. I may be off-balance, like the pendulum of a clock, but I'm going to start ticking! If a clock can work off-balance so can I!'

If I can get people to accept that much then the hard part – and the counselling – is over and we can get down to the fun bit: the therapy! (And if I can't do it I will find someone who can. The good thing about running a centre for people with MS that is part of a health club is that there are always plenty of others around to help if I can't. None of them are trained counsellors of course – I'm not myself – but most of them have been through many of the same problems and are usually more than happy to lend a friendly ear. A problem shared is a problem halved it has been said, rightly I think, and especially if it is with other people with MS. They are the very best type of counsellors: people like you who have found a way forward.)

The important point is this: you will almost certainly find that once you are looking at the problem in a positive light everyone starts to help you more. They become more constructive in their help and advice instead of being simply sympathetic. Sympathy is nice but it doesn't change anything. Asking someone to help by doing something positive for you makes everyone feel better: you feel less helpless and your helpers feel less pressurised. Actions, after all, speak louder than words!

Physical treatments

Even though the talking comes first, and can do a lot to help lift depression on its own in some people, physical therapies of various sorts are very helpful for those who find it hard to talk. So I look to start them as soon as possible on

- diet and nutrition
- massage and aromatherapy
- reflexology.

■ Diet and nutrition

Eating your way out of depression is very much a matter of eating for any condition: it means having a nutritious and balanced diet regularly. Eat a wholefood diet, with lots of fresh fruit and vegetables (but make sure they are washed to remove pesticides and preservatives) and avoid sugar, chocolate and other refined carbohydrates, saturated and animals fats, tea, coffee and drinks high in caffeine such as colas, and all other junk foods. Alcohol may be relaxing initially but too much for too long can have the opposite effect. Eating regularly is also important. It prevents slumps in the level of blood sugar in the body and evens out energy 'highs' and 'lows'.

Note: Giving up all caffeine suddenly can cause withdrawal headaches and a drop in energy for up to 48 hours afterwards if intake is high. Either be prepared to work through this or cut down gradually. Herbal teas such as marjoram, mist, verbena and thyme make excellent replacements for tea and coffee in cases of depression.

Supplements for depression (*daily doses*)

Calcium	500mg
Magnesium	200-400mg
Vitamin B-complex	50mg
Zinc*	15mg
Vitamin C	up to 3g

* Zinc should be taken only in the form of zinc gluconate, zinc sulphate, amino chelate or zinc orotate. It is the amount of elemental (pure) zinc you take that is important and this should be clearly shown on the label.

■ Massage and aromatherapy

A firm massage around the neck area and across the shoulders is wonderfully comforting and reassuring as well as stress-relieving.

The ideal is to have someone do it to you, but it is possible – though not easy – to treat yourself if you prefer or have no choice in the matter.

The best way to massage for depression is to use aromatherapy oils. No two people's depression is quite the same (just as no two people's MS is the same) and the important thing is to choose the right oils for what you think is the particular cause or causes of your depression.

If you are unsure which oil or oils you need the best way to decide is to smell them. Go to a shop where they have samplers and select those you like the smell of. There is a good chance your sense of smell knows some-

> **The following oils are good for depression:**
>
> *A general antidepressant*
> Bergamot
>
> *As a sedative and antidepressant*
> Sandalwood and ylang ylang
>
> *To lift mood without sedating*
> Bergamot, geranium, melissa and rose
>
> *For depression linked to restlessness, irritability and insomnia*
> Chamomile, clary sage, and lavender
>
> *For depression with anxiety*
> Neroli
>
> *For increased confidence*
> Jasmine

thing you don't – and the fact that you like the smell can often be because it's the one you need. Remember, this preference will change from day to day, depending on your mood. That's normal too.

There are a number of ways of using the oils. You can mix them with a base oil such as grapeseed oil and simply rub them on yourself wherever you like, rather like a perfume, you can put a few drops in your bath (heaven!), you can put them in a room spray, on a light bulb before it gets hot or in special vapourisers you can buy especially for the purpose.

■ Reflexology

As we've seen earlier in this book, reflexology is extremely effective for most physical conditions but it is also an excellent relaxer and that makes it outstanding for depression. Anything that helps the body relax helps the mind also. The areas to concentrate on are shown in the diagram below.

Guide to treatment

Adrenals
To balance energy levels and regulate stress

Pituitary gland
To regulate hormone levels

Diaphragm/ Solar plexus
To relax and regulate breathing

Lungs
To relax breathing

Thyroid
To help balance metabolism

Toes
To help clear the head

Liver
To stimulate release of toxins (a cause of 'sluggish' feelings)

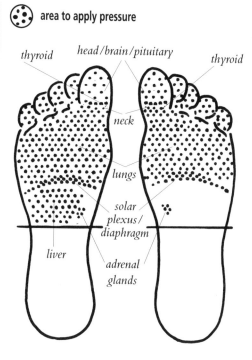

area to apply pressure

Reflexology points to relieve depression

Many of the tips and guidance on tiredness and fatigue in chapter 10 are helpful for depression so don't be afraid to make use of those you like the sound of or feel right to you. You are a better judge of how to treat yourself than you probably realize – and taking responsibility for yourself is the first step to getting on that road to recovery you want to be on.

Listen to your body and THINK POSITIVE!

postscript

Obviously my first concern in this book has been to offer anyone with MS clear and, hopefully, practical information that gives them positive benefit today – or, if not today, at least as soon as possible. But I am well aware that there are many people out there working to find ways of removing the scourage of MS completely.

If some process could be found, for example, that will repair the myelin and restore the proper signals to affected parts of the body I will be among the very first to welcome it and try it.

Among those dedicated researchers is someone I have worked with and got to know well over the years. Like me, Diana McGovern has MS and, like me also, wants desperately to help others. A few years ago she helped set up a project that is making great strides in the fight to find a cure for MS. It is called The Myelin Project.

The Myelin Project, or The British Trust for the Myelin Project to give it its full name, is an international charity whose single aim is to promote and accelerate research into how myelin might be restored. A unique non-profit partnership of top neurologists, researchers and interested lay people, the project has advanced to the point at which it claims to be just 'a step away' from success.

According to Diana, who is the project's unpaid secretary, working from their base in Edinburgh, Scotland, research has shown that transplantation of myelin-forming cells can form new myelin. That means that, in theory at least, myelin can be restored in people with MS. The research has shown that this is possible but it has only been tried so far on animals. It has not yet been tested on human tissue. So the next step is to try and do this.

The Myelin Project is establishing a dedicated Cell Culture Unit to develop the right sort of cells upon which to carry out the first human trials. This work is going on now and progress, reports Diana, is good. Of course it is likely to be some time yet before any results are known but at least progress is being made and there is hope that one day we may all get to hear the news some of us have waited many years to hear.

But so far we do not have that news. The odd person still pops up every now and then to claim they've found the miracle in a bottle of pop, make a bit of quick and easy money and disappear again without trace, but it never stands the test of time and we are never any better off. In the meantime, what are people with MS to do?

Well, that is what this book is all about. It may be that a miracle is around the corner but it is not here yet and until it is people with MS want something they can work with that will help them right away, now, today. That is why I have written this book.

Diana put it best in a recent letter to me. 'While I am working with the Myelin Project for the future,' she wrote, 'you are taking care of the present. Your work is essential for the well-being of fellow-sufferers, keeping them in the best possible shape for the time when our researchers come up with the treatment we all hope and pray for.'

I hope everyone reading this book does find it helpful in keeping them in the best possible shape pending the arrival of the cure. But if you would like to help the work of the project or know more about it, Diana invites you to write to her at:

The British Trust for The Myelin Project
4 Cammo Walk
Edinburgh EH4 8AN
Scotland.

It would be helpful if you would please enclose a stamped, self-addressed envelope – and say you read about it in this book!

home exercise

programme

The following section is a complete summary of my home exercise programme for people with MS. Based on the work of the Peto Institute for Conductive Education in Hungary, the exercises are all gentle toning and coordinating routines that anyone can do quite safely at home on their own (though a few may need the assistance of a helper else as well). Before you start, though, I recommend you read the following notes:

For best results

■ Each group of exercises can be done individually under the heading for the part of the body you want to exercise but I recommend that for best results you do all the exercises in any particular section in the order I show them.

■ For maximum effect read each exercise out loud before attempting it. I have found that doing this not only helps people take it in and understand it better but it also helps the brain to transmit the right message to the relevant groups of muscles.

■ Do each exercise to a count of five spoken out loud. Speaking the count out loud not only helps to find the right rhythm but regulates your breathing. Correct breathing is as important as doing the exercise correctly.

■ Make these exercises part of your everyday life.

home exercise programme

■ Note: *Many of the exercises described here do not appear in the main part of the book and vice versa. This is because the book features only a selection of the best exercises, most of which can be done in isolation from other exercises and are, if you like, supplementary to the exercises in Appendix A. The programme featured in this appendix works best if done as a complete routine, with one exercise following another in succession.*

Arm Exercises

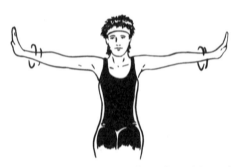

■ Exercise 1

Sit on an ordinary chair without arms to it and, with your back well supported by the back of the chair, hold your arms out to the side with the hands up and palms facing away from you as shown. Make small circles with each arm, moving the whole arm in a backwards rotation. Do this ten times. Repeat using, first, the left arm only and then the right arm.

■ Exercise 2

Still on the chair, sitting correctly, back straight, knees and feet slightly apart, hold your right arm up straight, fingers extended pointing at the ceiling. Make a large forwards circle. Do this ten times. Repeat with the left arm.

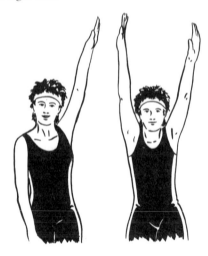

■ Exercise 3

Repeat exercise 2 with both arms together.

Back exercises

■ Exercise 1

You may need help for this exercise which is excellent for keeping the spine supple. Kneeling down on a flat, firm but comfortable surface, with your arms straight and your hands flat on the

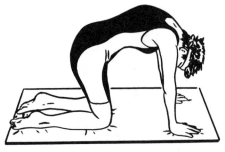

floor, arch your back at the same time as taking a deep breath and tucking your head down towards your chest. Breath out at the same time as dropping your back to the normal horizontal position and bringing your head right up so you are looking at the ceiling. Do this five times.

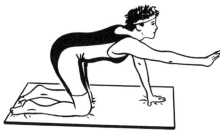

■ Exercise 2

Still on your hands and knees, lift your right arm up and in front of you to shoulder height. Do this to the count of five.

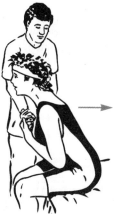

Repeat using your left arm. This exercise helps with balance.

■ Exercise 3

Sit on the edge of somewhere comfortable such as a bed, feet firmly on the floor, and with the assistance of a helper to hold onto, sway backwards and forwards as far as you possibly can.

home exercise programme

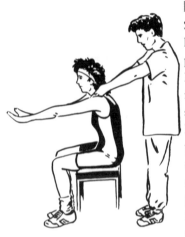

■ Exercise 4

Sitting on a sturdy chair ask your helper to stand behind you and place their hands on your shoulders. Holding your arms out straight in front of you as in the picture opposite, try and pull yourself forward, head up, while your helper pulls you gently back. Pull as hard as you can, even letting your feet come up off the floor if necessary. Hold the pull for five seconds before releasing. Do this five times. You must work closely with the helper on this exercise so that he or she gives enough resistance but not too much and learns how to increase the pull back as you get stronger.

■ Exercise 5

For this exercise you will need to stand in a doorway with your heels and backside against the doorframe and your forearms on a pillow or cushion on the opposite side. Now push into the pillow or cushion as hard as you can at the same time as pushing your bottom against the frame so that you are exerting pressure in two directions at once.

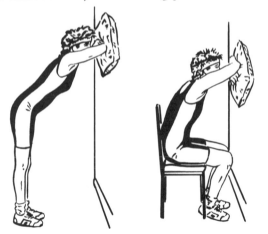

Increase the pressure gradually by increasing the amount of push. For those who have difficulty standing, sitting in a chair as in the diagram left will do just as well.

Back and leg exercises

■ Exercise 1

Kneeling somewhere firm but comfortable, lift your right leg straight up behind you to the count of five. Try and keep the leg straight and lift it as far up as pos-

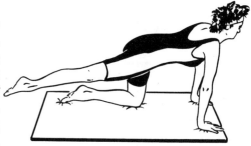

sible so that it is horizontal. Repeat with the left leg. Now try doing the same thing lifting alternate legs and arms (right leg, left arm, and left leg, right arm) at the same time. You will probably need someone to help you with this in case you topple over – which most people do at first! Do each exercise once each leg.

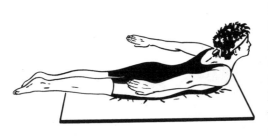

■ Exercise 2

Lie on your stomach with your arms stretched out in front of you and legs straight behind you. To the count of five bring your

right arm behind you, palm facing down and arm straight. Do the same thing with your left arm. Repeat with both arms at the same time and holding your head up.

Leg exercises

■ Exercise 1

Lie flat on your back on a firm, comfortable surface, legs straight (with toes up) and arms down by your sides. Relax. When you feel completely relaxed bend your right leg up to the count of five, making sure you

home exercise programme

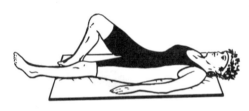

keep your foot on the floor. Hold that position for another count of five and then, to a further count of five, drop your leg slowly down again to the floor. Repeat with your left leg.

■ Exercise 2

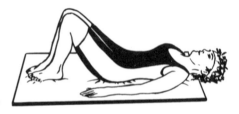

Continuing on from the above exercise, bend both legs up to the count of five and hold for another count of five. Now, again to a count of five, drop the right knee to the side and hold for a count of five. Do the same with the left knee so that both knees are as wide apart as possible. Hold for a count of five, bring both knees together and, to a final count of five, lower both legs to the ground.

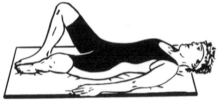

■ Exercise 3

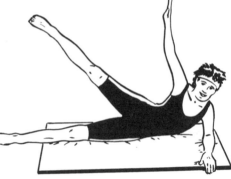

Roll over onto your left side with legs straight out and arms down by your side. Keeping the leg straight, lift your right leg and right arm together. Hold the position to the count of five and then lower both to another count of five. Still in that position pull both knees up to your stomach (as in the foetus position) and hold for a count of five. Return both legs and arms to their original position to another count of five. Roll over onto your right side and repeat the above with your left leg and arm.

■ Exercise 4

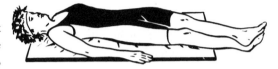

On your back now, move the right leg out to the side – making sure to keep it straight – to the count of five. Keeping the right leg out, do the same with the left leg. Both legs should now be wide apart. Now move the right leg to the count of five so that the right ankle lies across the left ankle. Hold for a count of five and return the right leg to the wide open position to another count of five. Repeat crossing the left leg over the right, always counting to five for each movement. Complete the exercise by returning both legs to the closed position to a count of five.

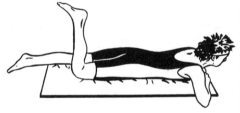

■ Exercise 5

Lying flat on your stomach, bend your right leg up behind you (again to five). Hold for five and lower to five. Repeat using first your left leg and then both legs together.

■ Exercise 6

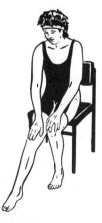

Sitting in a sturdy chair or wheelchair, back straight, feet flat on the floor, bottom slightly forward on the seat, move your right leg out, foot still on the floor, so that the leg is straight out in front of you. Keeping your heel on the floor, lift your foot upwards to point your toes at the ceiling to the count of five. Do this five times and then bring the leg back to the normal sitting position. Repeat using your left leg. Now do the same again with both legs together. Get someone to help hold your foot straight if you can't do it yourself. This exercise strengthens the front of the lower leg, foot and ankle.

Exercise 7

Sit back into the chair with shoulders back, legs straight, knees slightly apart and both feet on the ground. To the count of five, lift your right leg so that it is straight out in front of you in a horizontal position. Hold it there for a count of five before bringing it back down to another count of five. Repeat with your left leg. To increase resistance you can add small weights to your ankles. Hold onto the chair seat if it makes it easier.

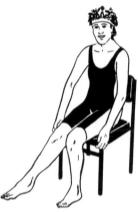

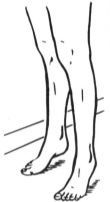

Exercise 8

Standing behind a sturdy chair and holding firmly onto it for support, raise and lower yourself using only your toes as in the illustration on the left. Do it 15 times. Make sure you keep your back straight and your knees slightly bent when you do this exercise.

Exercise 9

Still standing behind a sturdy chair and holding onto it for support (or you could use any other firm hold at the same height), squat down so that your knees are at right angles and at 'hip width' apart before coming back up again. Try and keep your heels flat on the floor if you can but it doesn't matter if you find you have to lift them slightly. Do this exercise ten times. See diagram at the top of the next page.

Exercise 10

It's best to wear light shoes for this exercise and you'll also need a large book, house brick or something of a similar width. See diagram

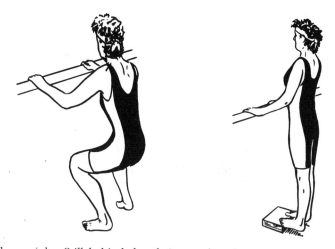

above right. Still behind the chair, stand with just your toes on the book or brick and your heels on the floor. Stand straight up and keep your backside out. You should feel a 'pull' in the back of your legs and calf muscles. This is a very effective muscle-stretching exercise and you should try and hold the position for as long as possible.

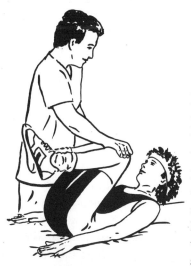

■ Exercise 11

You will need a helper with this exercise. Lie on your back with your knees pulled up to your chest and get your helper to push against your knees while you try to push your knees as hard as you can away from you. You should feel your face become hot with the exertion. Hold this position for five seconds. Repeat five times. Now reverse the situation, so your helper pulls your knees away while you try to draw them up as hard as you can. Hold for five seconds. Do it five times.

home exercise programme

■ Exercise 12

This exercise is known as the 'pelvic tilt'. Lie on a firm, comfortable surface such the floor or a bed with your knees bent up and feet flat on the surface. Keeping your shoulders and feet on the floor or bed, lift your backside up, clenching in the muscles and holding for five seconds. Relax and repeat five times.

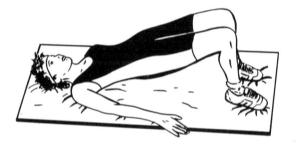

■ Exercise 13

This one is really fun! Stand at the foot of a bed and fall backwards onto the bed in a control fall. Roll your knees up to your chest as you fall and at the end of the

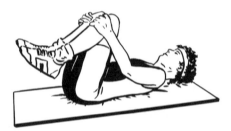

roll immediately roll back again to stand on your feet at the foot of the bed again. Do this at least ten times a day. If you're anything like me, you'll want to do it a hundred times a day!

Coordination exercises

■ Exercise 1

Sit in a chair a little forward in the seat with both feet firmly on the ground and clenched fists on each knee with the thumbs pointing up. Lift the right thumb off the knee and bring it down to meet the thumb on the left knee by swinging the right arm in an arc behind you as if doing the 'front crawl' in swimming. Return the right hand to the right knee doing the same movement in reverse. Do each

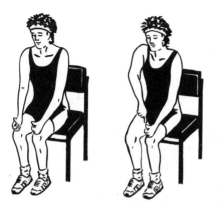

movement to the count of five. Repeat the whole exercise using each of the fingers in turn (the right index finger to the left index finger and so on). Once you've done all the fingers and the thumb of the right hand do the whole exercise again, this time swinging the left hand to meet the right hand.

Finally, repeat the entire process with your eyes closed!

■ Exercise 2

Still sitting as for exercise 1 (with clenched fists on each knee with the thumbs pointing up) bring the right thumb up to the point of the chin and return it to the right knee. Then bring the same thumb up to touch the point

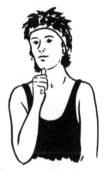

of your nose and back again. Now change the action to bring the inside of your right wrist up to touch your forehead and back to your knee. Keep the fist clenched and the thumb pointing up. Repeat the process using each finger on the right hand in turn, touching your forehead with the inside of your wrist between each one. Repeat the whole thing using your left hand, starting with the thumb again. Now do it all again with both hands but this time keeping your eyes closed.

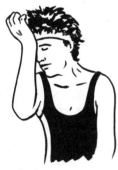

■ Exercise 3

You will need a thin stick or knitting needle for this really excellent coordination routine. Sit down with the stick or needle on the floor in front of you. Bend down and, to the count of five, pick the stick/needle up with both hands using only the fingertips and thumbs and keeping both arms straight. Holding the stick/needle between the thumb and index finger of the right hand and the thumb

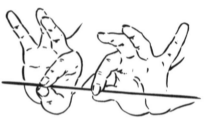

and index finger of the left hand. Now making sure you keep the thumb in the same position hold the stick with the same finger of both hands in turn, rather like playing the piano. So after holding the stick with the thumb/index finger of each hand hold it between the thumb/middle finger, thumb/third finger and finally thumb/little finger. Then return through the fingers from the little finger back to the index finger. Do this five times. Now do the exercise with just one hand, starting with your right hand and then the left. Finally, do the whole sequence again with your eyes closed. It may seem hard – and usually is at first – but you'll get better. It can become a lot of fun too!

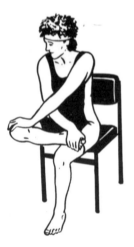

■ Exercise 4

This is a good ankle-strengthening exercise. Sit on a chair with both feet firmly on the ground. Bend down and, holding the inside of the right ankle with the right hand, lift it up and place it on the left knee, resting the ankle on the knee and keeping the left leg firmly on the floor. Place the left hand on top of the right knee keeping the right hand on the right ankle. Push the knee down five times. Take the hands off the knee and rotate the foot ten times clockwise followed by ten times anti-clockwise. Do this unaided if possible. Repeat five to ten times. If you can't do this unaided rotate the foot yourself with your left hand. Repeat the exercise using your left leg over your right.

■ Exercise 5

Sitting on the chair, bend your right leg up and put your foot onto the chair. Do this unaided if possible. Hold your foot on the chair to the count of five and then lower it again, also to the count of five. Repeat using the left leg and then both legs, again to the count of five. You can clasp your knees with your arms if necessary to keep them up.

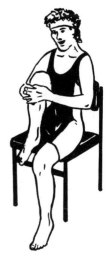

■ *Most of the exercises in this Appendix are also demonstrated in my video 'MS – A Home Video Programme', available direct from Under Pressure Publications at £17.95 including post and packing.*

the 'leaky gut' connection

What 'leaky gut' is

Leaky gut, or 'leaky gut syndrome' as it is more usually called, is a condition in which the delicate inner lining or mucous membrane of the intestines is damaged, usually as a result of inflammation caused by infection or chronic stress, so allowing various toxins to 'leak' into the bloodstream where they can cause a wide range of illnesses and other problems.

The condition is described medically as 'intestinal permeability' but so wide is the range of problems some experts now believe the condition can cause they are starting to call it 'leaky gut syndromes', in the plural.

Among serious chronic diseases it is believed it can cause, trigger or accelerate are arthritis, various skin complaints (such as acne, eczema and psoriasis), irritable bowel syndrome (IBS), Aids, chronic fatigue sundrome, hepatitis, cystic fibrosis and cancer. My belief is that MS may be another.

The link with MS

The condition is, I believe, strongly implicated in MS not only because many of the symptoms of MS – such as muscle spasms, inability to exercise for long, poor memory and concentration, shallow breathing, fatigue, depression, diarrhoea and constipation, food allergies, and pain in the joints and muscles are those associated with leaky gut syndrome but also because many of the factors that I consider can cause MS are those behind leaky gut syndrome too. As detailed in chapter 2, these include:

- stress
- trauma and shock
- crash dieting and/or fasting
- viral infections
- yeast overgrowth *(candidiasis)*.

In essence, I believe that people with MS are prone to leaky gut because of a characteristic deficiency in nutrients important for the proper working of the digestive process made worse by a corresponding weakness of tissue in the intestines and the muscles that control them.

Various researchers, particularly in America, have theorized about toxins entering the bloodstream through the intestines as a possible cause of MS – notably Dr Robert Soll – but I may be the first to see the possible link between MS and the growing problem of 'leaky gut'.

My own researches have shown stress and emotional trauma to be common among people with MS – and often such stress itself results in dietary deficiencies and low nutritional intake. Stress, for example, reduces stomach acid and this can lead to bacterial overgrowth through a reduction of the vital B vitamin biotin. Stress also reduces the amount of vitamin B12 in the body – and we know that B12 is notoriously deficient in people with MS.

My case also holds up if we look at the theory that MS is an auto-immune disease caused by the body failing to recognise its own tissue and attacking it as 'foreign' (see chapter 2). A leaky gut allows toxins into the bloodstream that could, in susceptible people, cause just the sort of 'auto-immune' reaction that damages the myelin sheath. Experts claim that in people with a different susceptibility it can cause arthritis so it is surely just as possible that MS could be yet another outcome. Again, we know that stress plays a part in auto-immune disease too.

The gluten and fat connection

People with MS seem to have a particular sensitivity to gluten, a 'sticky' protein found in grains such as wheat, rye, oats and barley, and this is why many people with MS are recommended a gluten-free diet. Sensivity to gluten can cause inflammation of the delicate lining of the gut wall resulting in malabsorption of food. This can lead to any number of illnesses, the most serious being coeliac disease in which the small intestine fails to absorb almost any of the nutrients, including fats, the body needs to survive. The disease is commonest among children but a milder version in adults is known as 'sprue'.

The normal treatment is simply to avoid all foods containing gluten. Foods high in gluten are bread, pasta, cakes and biscuits (cookies) – and so it is easy to see why many people find this a particularly hard diet to keep to. But there is now evidence that eating lots of oily fish such as tuna, sardines, herrings and mackerel can help. Oily fish contain high amounts of a particular sort of essential fatty acid (EFA) that appears to reinforce the gut lining. Another good source of this EFA, known as the 'omega-3' family of EFAs, is dark green leafy vegetables. Also helpful is a second type of EFA known as 'omega-6'. This is found in sunflower and safflower seeds, legumes (peas and beans) and breast milk.

EFAs can be taken in capsule form as food supplements – omega-3 as fish or marine oil concentrate and omega-6 as oil of evening primrose (EPO), borage/starflower or blackcurrant.

Note that this recommendation does not contradict that other very important dietary advice in MS not to eat animal fat. Animal fat is saturated fat and is very different from EFAs. Saturated fat interferes with and 'blocks' the good 'polyunsaturated' (PUFAs) and 'monounsaturated' fats (MUFAs) we need to maintain a healthy gut.

So by all means cut down on, and preferably cut out, animal fat from your diet but do not reduce your intake of oily fish, dark green leafy vegetables or sunflower seeds.

So whether the prime cause is stress or nutritional deficiency or both interacting (which I think is the most likely) I now believe these factors can produce a vicious cycle of cause-and-effect that may have a significant role to play in aggravating the effects of MS – *if not, perhaps, even causing them in the first place.*

Can you help?

At the moment, exciting though it is, all that I have said about the links between leaky gut syndrome and MS is in the realms of speculation. I believe I have uncovered something of significance but I do not know for certain. Investigation is at an early stage and much more work needs to be done to refine both the theory and practice.

I have recently set up a foundation – The Susie Cornell Foundation – to further this and my other work and I would be delighted to hear from anyone, individual, organisation or company, either with experience of the problem or who might be interested in working with me to advance both our general understanding of the problem and its safe and affective treatment.

Please write to me at the address on page 184.

taking food supplements

In the main part of the book I tell you what food supplements to take for various problems and how much to take. But there is more to supplement taking than simply swallowing the right dose of the right vitamin or mineral. For example, when you take them is also important, and for how long and with what.

Though taking the right dose of the right supplement will always help, the benefits may not be as good as they could and should be unless you follow a few simple rules. So to help you make sure you get the most from food supplements here are my ten top tips for effective supplement taking:

Top tips for taking supplements effectively

■ 1 Always take vitamins and minerals with food. If you can't or don't want to swallow them with a meal, make sure you take them no earlier than 15 minutes before or 15 minutes after.

■ 2 Take your supplements every day without fail. Taking supplements irregularly doesn't work.

■ 3 B vitamins (there are over 12 known B vitamins and more are being discovered) should not be taken separately from each other. All B vitamins work synergistically – that is, they work together in combination – and so it is always best to take them as a 'complex', even if you only need, say, B12.

■ 4 Don't take B vitamins or B complex late at night, especially if you have difficulty sleeping.

■ 5 Individual minerals should not be taken in isolation so always take a B complex or multivitamin if you are taking individual minerals such as zinc.

■ 6 Taking multiminerals in the evening can help you sleep.

■ 7 If you are taking more than one B complex or vitamin C tablet or capsule a day try to split them up so that you take half the dose at breakfast and the other half at lunch.

■ 8 Avoid 'ferric' forms of iron if you are taking iron supplements for anaemia (iron deficiency) and always take vitamin C as well.

■ 9 Don't persevere with a given dose of supplements for a particular condition longer than about three months if you are not seeing positive changes. Go along to a properly-qualified nutritional therapist and ask for advice. See a therapist as soon as possible if you experience anything at any time that makes you feel anxious or unwell.

■ What to do if there are side-effects

Food supplements are nutrients, not drugs. So provided you stick to the levels recommended the only side-effects are likely to be beneficial ones such as increased energy, improved mental alertness and greater resistance to disease. But just occasionally a few people do react even to the recommended dose levels. Though such reactions are not serious in the way reactions to some drugs can be it is worth noting the possible reasons and what to do about it.

One reason for side-effects is taking too many supplements with too little food. Another is an allergic reaction to something in the supplement such as yeast. A few supplements can be toxic if taken in too high a dose or at the wrong time (such as during pregnancy). Vitamin A (but not beta carotene), zinc, iron and selenium are examples of supplements that can be toxic but the doses have to be very high indeed – far higher than any of the doses recommended by manufacturers – for there to be any real danger. Again, take advice if you are not sure.

taking food supplements

Problems of allergic reaction or sensitivity to ingredients can be solved by stopping the supplements altogether and trying to isolate the culprit by a process of elimination. Wait four days and then introduce just one of the supplements you were taking. Take it on its own for four days. If there is no reaction introduce another for another four days and note how you feel. If there is still no reaction take a third, and so on until you have either identified the guilty party or the problem you thought you had is no longer there. It is surprising how often the original problem can go away using this method.

Another occasional phenomenon with food supplements worth pointing out is the 'getting worse before you get better' syndrome. Stoking up your body with nutrients it has lacked and desperately needed can stimulate a process known by natural therapists as 'detoxification' or 'cleansing'. A detoxifying or 'cleansing reaction' can make you feel slightly worse in the early stages as the body learns to adapt and starts to get rid of the poisons it has accumulated over the years from pollution, a poor diet, lack of exercise and generally unhealthy living.

This is a normal and natural process and is nothing to be unduly alarmed about. It is usually subsides within about a month and you start to feel the full benefits of a healthier body. If for any reason, though, the symptoms do not subside or you develop symptoms that you can't explain and that worry you have no hesitation in seeing a nutritional therapist for advice.

■ How long to take supplements

The effect of supplements is cumulative over a long time, usually years. Supplements, as I've already said, are not drugs so you should not expect any overnight miracles. But though long-term benefits take years to build, improvements should normally start to be felt within about three months. Surveys have found that this is the average time for benefits such as improved energy, mental alertness, skin condition, emotional tranquillity and overall well-being to show themselves. These improvements should continue and remain as long as you are following the right programme for you. If they don't show or don't continue it is, again, best to see a therapist for advice.

But whether or not they show or continue it is sensible to think in terms of seeing a therapist every three months for a proper assessment, particularly in the early stages of treatment. Individual needs change and your need for nutrients is likely to change as you become healthier. The same applies if you suffer a relapse or are ill for any reason. The need for optimum nutrition increases dramatically whenever you are under stress and strain, going through a crisis or working especially hard. A good therapist will be able to advise on the right adjustments to be made to your programme to keep you healthy and moving forward. So remember the three-month rule.

Finally, don't be reluctant to see a properly qualified nutritionist if you are at all unsure about the exact dose or combination of vitamins and minerals to take. But if you don't want to see a specialist and would rather treat yourself remember that it is usually best to opt for a multi-vitamin and multi-mineral formula from a reputable supplier than try to work out your own programme.

Remember also that it is best to have a proper nutritional analysis done before starting any programme, especially before taking mineral supplements, and that's why I recommend having a hair mineral test done. Any good nutritionist will be able to arrange this for you.

Free nutritional advice for people with MS is available in the UK and Europe from Lamberts Healthcare (Nature's Best) on 01892 552119/55120-1. For details of where to write to Lamberts Healthcare see the following page.

taking food supplements

Suppliers of supplements

Leading brands of supplements are available from most pharmacies and healthfood stores. Leading brand names in Britain include Biocare, Blackmores, Quest Vitamins, Solgar, Larkhall Healthcare and Nature's Best. Nature's Best, a division of Lamberts Healthcare, are the only company so far to offer a special deal for people with MS. Sufferers in Europe, including the UK and Eire, can contact them at the address below.

> **Nature's Best**
> 1 Lamberts Road
> Tunbridge Wells
> Kent TN2 3EQ, UK.
> Tel 01892 552120

Nature's Best specializes in the quick and efficient mail order supply of the food supplements mentioned in this book. The company also offers people with MS free supplements up to the value of £15 and 10% discount on all subsequent orders on production of a doctor's certificate confirming diagnosis.

resources

Courses for therapists and carers

A number of the treatments described in this book need to be carried out by qualified therapists for maximum benefit and safety. Training courses and seminars for professional healthcarers who would like to know more about both the theory and practice involved in any of the therapies mentioned are available through the Under Pressure School of Natural Therapy

Doctors, nurses, aromatherapists, nutritionists, massage therapists, reflexologists, physiotherapists and physical therapists are particularly welcome to apply. For further details contact me, Susie Cornell, at:

Under Pressure School of Natural Therapy
P O Box 1270
Chelmsford
Essex CM2 6BQ
United Kingdom

Fax 01245 252280

The Susie Cornell Foundation

The Susie Cornell Foundation has been set up to help people with MS and those who assist them, whether family or carers, through research, treatment and education.

■ Research

The Foundation encourages and promotes new areas of research into the causes and treatment of MS, especially those treatments that concentrate on safe, gentle and effective therapies such as natural therapy, nutrition and counselling.

■ Treatment

The Foundation assists those who cannot afford it to have the treatment recommended by Susie Cornell.

■ Education

The Foundation organises and promotes workshops, seminars and conferences to teach the treatments recommended by Susie Cornell for MS to as wide an audience as possible, as well as publishes a range of self-help books, videos, audio-tapes and leaflets for the same purpose.

Further information on the Foundation can be obtained by writing, preferably with a self-addressed, stamped envelope, to:

The Secretary
The Susie Cornell Foundation
PO Box 1270
Chelmsford
Essex CM2 6BQ, UK.

Useful organizations

■ International

International Federation of Multiple Sclerosis Societies
10 Heddon Street
London W1R 7JL, UK.
Tel 0171-734 9120
Fax 0171-287 2587.

■ Australasia

MS Society of New Zealand
7th Floor, Rossmore House
123 Molesworth Street
PO Box 2627
Wellington
New Zealand.
Tel 644 499 4677
Fax 644 499 4675.

National MS Society of Australia
Private Bag Q1000
QVB Post Office
Sydney
New South Wales 2000
Australia.
Tel 612 287 2929
Fax 612 287 2987.

■ North America

Feldenkrais Guild
8718 West 110th Street,
Suite 140
Overland Park
Kansas 66210, USA
Tel 913 345 1141

MS Society of Canada
Suite 820
250 Bloor St East
Toronto
Ontario M4W 3P9, Canada.
Tel 416 922 6065
Fax 416 922 7538.

National MS Society
205 East 42 Street
New York
New York 10017 5700, USA.
Tel 212 986 3420
Fax 212 986 7981.

North American Society of Teachers of the Alexander Technique
PO Box 3992
Champagne
Illinois 61826-3992, USA.

■ Southern Africa

MS Society of Zimbabwe
PO Box 8214
Causeway
Harare
Zimbabwe.
Tel 263 796 957.

South African National MS Society
295 Villiers Road, Walmer
Port Elizabeth 6070,South Africa.
Tel/fax 4151 2900.

■ Europe (inc UK and Eire)

Association of MS Therapy Centres (Scotland)
Unit 1, Saxbone Centre
Howmoss Crescent
Kirk Hill Industrial Estate
Dyce
Aberdeen AB2 0GN, Scotland
Tel 01224 771105

Federation of Multiple Sclerosis Therapy Centres
Unit 4
Murdock Road
Bedford MK41 7PD, UK.
Tel 01234 325781

A network of 67 self-governing local patient support centres covering Great Britain and Ireland set up in 1993. The Federation also represents both the Northern Association and the Scottish Association of MS Therapy Centres.

Feldenkrais Method
28a Hampstead High Street
London NW3 1QA.

Meir Schneider's Self-Healing Approach
c/o Pat Sawyer
15 Haggerston Road
Borehamwood
Herts WD6 4BU, UK.
Tel 0181 953 9504

MS Research Charitable Trust
Spirella Building
Letchworth
Hertfordshire SG6 4ET, UK.
Tel 01462 675613

Multiple Sclerosis Resource Centre
4a Chapel Hill
Stansted
Essex CM24 8AG, UK.
Tel 01279 817101
Fax 01279 647179

Multiple Sclerosis Society of Great Britain & Northern Ireland
25 Effie Road
London SW6 1YZ, UK.
Tel 0171-736 6267
Fax 0171-736 9861

Multiple Sclerosis Society of Ireland
2 Sandymount Green
Dublin 4, Eire.
Tel 0126 94599
Fax 0126 93746

Multiple Sclerosis Training, Education and Research Trust (MUSTER)
PO Box 122
Berkhamsted
Herts HP4 3HA, UK.
Fax 01442 870792

MUSTER was set up in 1994, partly in succession to Action & Research in Multiple Sclerosis (ARMS).

MS Under Pressure (Susie Cornell)
PO Box 1270
Chelmsford
Essex CM2 6BQ, UK.
Fax 01245 252280

National Institute for Conductive Education
Cannon Hill House
Russell Road
Moseley
Birmingham B13 8RD, UK.
Tel 0121-449 1569
Fax 0121-449 1611

Northern Association of MS Therapy Centres
c/o GEC Alston
PO Box 132
Westinghouse Road
Trafford Park
Manchester M60 1GE, UK.
Tel 0161-872 3422

Peto Institute for Conductive Education
Kutvolgyi ut 6, 1125
Budapest X11, Hungary.

Society of Teachers of the Alexander Technique
20 London House
266 Fulham Road
London SW10 9EL, UK.
Tel 0171-351 0828

The British Trust for the Myelin Project
4 Cammo Walk
Edinburgh EH4 8AN,
Scotland.
Tel 0131 339 1316

Yoga for Health Foundation
Ickwell Bury
Biggleswade
Bedfordshire
SG18 9EF, UK.
Tel 0767 627271

Further reading

You might find the following books useful if you'd like more detail or background on the information in this handbook. Please refer direct to the publishers or authors themselves if you would like copies of the books or of any of the material in them.

All Day Energy, Kathryn Marsden *(Bantam Books, UK, 1995)*
Aromatherapy: An A–Z, Patricia Davis *(C W Daniel, UK, 1988)*
Asthma and Beyond, Paul Sherwood *(Arrow Books, UK, 1995)*
Coping with MS, Cynthia Benz *(Macdonald -Optima, UK, 1988)*
Digestive Enzymes, Jeffery Bland *(Keats Publishing, USA, 1983)*
Fitness Programming and Physical Disability, ed Patricia D Miller *(Human Kinetics, USA, 1995)*
Food Combining for Health, Doris Grant & Jean Joice (Thorsons, UK, 1984)
Getting Firm, ed Charles L Mee *(Time-Life Books, USA, 1987)*
Immune Power, Jennifer Meek *(Optima, UK, 1990)*
Mass Immunisation, Trevor Gunn *(Cutting Edge Publications, USA, 1992)*
Multiple Sclerosis – The Self-Help Guide, Judy Graham *(Thorsons, UK, 1992)*
Native Nutrition, Ronald Schmid *(Healing Arts, USA, 1994)*
Nutritional Medicine, Stephen Davies & Alan Stewart *(Pan Books, UK, 1987)*
Planning for a Healthy Baby, Belinda Barnes & Suzanna Gail Bradley *(Vermilion Books, UK, 1994)*
Raw Energy, Leslie and Susannah Kenton *(Vermilion Books, UK, 1994)*
Self-Healing, Meir Schneider *(Arkana-Penguin, UK/USA, 1989)*
Shiatsu and Stretching, Toru Namikoshi *(Japan Publications, Japan/ USA, 1985)*
The Amino Revolution, Robert Erdmann and Meirion Jones *(Century Hutchinson, UK, 1989)*
The Back and Beyond, Paul Sherwood *(Arrow Books, UK, 1992)*
The Better Diet Book, Lynne McTaggart *(Wallace Press, UK, 1995)*
The Heart Revolution, Paul Sherwood *(Arrow Books, UK, 1994)*
The Reflexology Handbook, Laura Norman and Thomas Cowan *(Piatkus Books, UK, 1988)*
The Vitamin Bible, Earl Mindell *(Arlington Books, USA, 1994)*
The Natural Way with MS, Richard Thomas *(Element Books, 1995)*
Touch and Stretch, Carolan Evans *(Mackenzie Publishing, UK, 1991)*
Yoga for the Disabled, Howard Kent *(Thorsons, UK, 1985)*
You Don't Have to Feel Unwell, Robin Needes *(Gateway Books, UK, 1994)*

index